W9-DDJ-220

FIRST AID FOR THE

USMLE STEP 1

A STUDENT TO **UPDATED FOR 1996** STUDENT GUIDE

VIKAS BHUSHAN, MD
University of California, San Francisco, Class of 1991
University of California, Los Angeles, Resident in Diagnostic Radiology

TAO LE
University of California, San Francisco
School of Medicine, Class of 1996

CHIRAG AMIN
University of Miami
School of Medicine, Class of 1996

APPLETON & LANGE
Stamford, Connecticut

Notice: The authors and publisher of this volume have taken care that the information and recommendations contained herein are accurate and compatible with standards generally accepted at the time of publication. Nevertheless, it is difficult to ensure that all the information given is entirely accurate for all circumstances. The publisher disclaims any liability, loss, or damage incurred as a consequence, directly or indirectly, of the use or application of any of the contents of this volume.

Copyright © 1996 by Appleton & Lange
A Simon & Schuster Company
First edition copyright © 1989, 1990 by Vikas Bhushan, Jeffrey Hansen, and Edward Hon
Copyright © 1991, 1992, 1993 by Appleton & Lange

Information from the following titles was incorporated into Section II: Database of High-Yield Facts, and was used with permission: Katzung BG (editor), *Basic & Clinical Pharmacology,* 6th ed., Appleton & Lange, 1995; Goldman HH, *Review of General Psychiatry,* 5th ed., Appleton & Lange, 1992; Ganong WF, *Review of Medical Physiology,* 15th ed., Appleton & Lange, 1991; Levinson W, *Medical Microbiology and Immunology: Examination and Board Review,* 3rd ed., Appleton & Lange, 1994; Chandrasoma P. *Concise Pathology,* 1st ed. Appleton & Lange, 1991; Costanzo L, *BRS Physiology,* 1st ed., Williams & Wilkins, 1995. The diagram on p. 93 was adapted from *N Engl J Med* 1983; **309:**288. The diagram on p. 125 was adapted from *Curr Opin Infect Dis* 1992; **5:**214.

All rights reserved. This book, or any parts thereof, may not be used or reproduced in any manner without written permission. For information, address Appleton & Lange, Four Stamford Plaza, PO Box 120041, Stamford, Connecticut 06912-0041.

96 97 98 / 10 9 8 7 6 5 4 3 2 1

Prentice Hall International (UK) Limited, *London*
Prentice Hall of Australia Pty. Limited, *Sydney*
Prentice Hall of Canada, Inc., *Toronto*
Prentice Hall Hispanoamericana, S.A., *Mexico*
Prentice Hall of India Private Limited, *New Delhi*
Prentice Hall of Japan, Inc., *Tokyo*
Simon & Schuster Asia Pte. Ltd., *Singapore*
Editora Prentice Hall do Brasil Ltda., *Rio de Janeiro*
Prentice Hall, *Upper Saddle River, New Jersey*

ISBN: 0-8385-2593-8

ISBN 0-8385-2597-0

Acquisitions Editors: John Dolan and Marinita Timban
Production Services: Rainbow Graphics, Inc.
Editorial Consultant: Andrea Fellows

To the contributors to this and future editions, who took time to share their knowledge, insight, and humor for the benefit of students.

&

To our families, friends and loved ones, who endured and assisted in the task of assembling this guide.

1996 Contributors

TAEJOON AHN
Contributing Author, High-Yield Facts
University of California, San Francisco, Class of 1997

ALIREZA ATRI
Contributing Author, High-Yield Facts
University of California, San Francisco, Class of 1997

ROSS BERKELEY
Contributing Author, High-Yield Facts
University of California, San Francisco, Class of 1997

CHRISTINE PHAM
Contributing Editor, Review Books
University of California, San Francisco, Class of 1997

JUDY SHIH
Contributing Author, High-Yield Facts
University of California, San Francisco, Class of 1997

DAVID STEENSMA
Contributing Author, High-Yield Facts
University of Chicago-Pritzker, Class of 1996

1996 Associate Contributors

ANTHONY GLASER, MD, PhD
Resident in Family Medicine
Medical University of South Carolina

KAMBIZ KOSARI
University of California, San Francisco, Class of 1997

MICHAEL RIZEN
University of California, San Francisco, Class of 1996

GARY ULANER
Stanford University, Class of 2000

1996 Faculty Reviewers

DEPARTMENT OF ANATOMY
University of California, San Francisco

WILLIAM GANONG, MD
Lange Professor of Physiology Emeritus
University of California, San Francisco

BERTRAM KATZUNG, MD, PhD
Professor of Pharmacology
University of California San Francisco

WARREN LEVINSON, MD, PhD
Professor of Microbiology and Immunology
University of California, San Francisco

HENRY SANCHEZ, MD
Assistant Clinical Professor of Pathology
University of California, San Francisco

VIJAY YAJNIK, PhD
Consultant Molecular Biologist
New York University, Class of 1996

Contents

Preface to the 1996 Edition

With the 1996 edition of *First Aid for the USMLE Step 1,* we continue our commitment to providing students with the most useful and up-to-date preparation guide for the USMLE Step 1. The 1996 edition represents a major revision in many ways and includes:

- Revisions and new material based on student experience with the June and September 1995 administrations of the USMLE Step 1.
- A revised and updated guide to efficient exam preparation, including new Step 1 statistics as well as new study and test-taking strategies.
- USMLE advice geared toward international medical graduates and osteopathic medical students.
- Over 800 frequently tested facts and useful mnemonics, including more than 90 new entries and 220 expanded entries with many new integrative diagrams and tables.
- An updated listing of over 150 high-yield study topics that highlight key areas of basic science and clinical material emphasized on the USMLE Step 1.
- A completely revised, in-depth guide to more than 175 basic science review and sample examination books, based on a random national survey of thousands of third-year medical students across the country. Includes over 30 new books and software titles.

The 1996 edition would not have been possible without student and faculty feedback and suggestions. We invite students and faculty to continue sharing their thoughts and ideas to help us improve *First Aid for the USMLE Step 1.* (*See* How to Contribute, p. xv, and User Survey, p. xxiii.)

Los Angeles   Vikas Bhushan
San Francisco   Tao Le
Miami   Chirag Amin

November 1995

Foreword

The purpose of *First Aid for the USMLE Step 1: A Student-to-Student Guide* is to help medical students and foreign medical graduates review the basic medical sciences and prepare for the United States Medical Licensing Examination, Step 1 (USMLE Step 1). Preparing for this examination can be a stressful, difficult, and costly task. This book helps students make the most of their limited time, money, and energy. As is often the case in medical school, we found that the best advice a student can receive is from other medical students. We also recognized that certain basic science topics and details are "popular" and appear frequently on examinations. With this in mind, *First Aid for the USMLE Step 1* was started in 1989.

As we studied for the NBME Part I, we examined and evaluated scores of review books and thousands of sample questions. We kept track of useful study strategies, frequently tested facts, and helpful mnemonics through a simple computer database. The printed database was first distributed to the medical school class of 1992 at the University of California, San Francisco (UCSF). The next year, a revised edition was self-published under the name *High-Yield Basic Science Boards Review: A Student-to-Student Guide.* This guide was distributed to the UCSF class of 1993 and to numerous faculty and medical students at various institutions.

The title reflects the potential value of this book as the "first" one to get before buying others, and the fact that boards examinations are stressful and unpleasant experiences that students may "aid" each other in overcoming. We feel that this study guide provides a unique, pragmatic approach to the USMLE Step 1 and that it contains useful components not found in current boards review material. *First Aid for the USMLE Step 1* has three major sections:

Section I: Guide to Efficient Exam Preparation is a compilation of general student advice and study strategies for taking the USMLE Step 1.

Section II: Database of High-Yield Facts contains short descriptions of frequently tested facts and concepts as well as mnemonics and diagrams to facilitate learning. It includes a unique summary of subject-by-subject examination emphases as estimated by students who have recently taken the examination.

Section III: Database of Basic Science Review Books is designed to save students time and money by identifying high-quality, reasonably priced review and sample examination books and software. The comments and ratings are based on our analyses and on a nationwide random sampling of third-year medical students.

First Aid for the USMLE Step 1 is not designed to be a comprehensive text or the sole study source for the USMLE Step 1; it is meant as a **guide** to one's preparation for the USMLE Step 1. The material in this book has been written to strengthen one's familiarity with a large number of topics in a short, fact-based review. The authors do not advocate blindly memorizing the lists of facts, and we hope medical students realize that memorization cannot replace an understanding of the concepts that underlie these key points.

Entries in *First Aid for the USMLE Step 1* originated from hundreds of students, foreign medical graduates, and faculty members, who synthesized the facts, notes, and mnemonics from a variety of textbooks, review books, lecture notes, and personal notes. We regret the inability to reference each individual fact or mnemonic owing to the diverse and often anecdotal sources. Though the material has been reviewed by faculty members and medical students, errors and omissions are inevitable. We urge readers to identify errors and suggest improvements. We regret that some students may find certain mnemonics trivializing or offensive. The mnemonics are meant solely as optional devices for learning.

The authors and Appleton & Lange intend to continue updating *First Aid for the USMLE Step 1* so that the book grows in quality and scope and continues to reflect the material covered on the USMLE Step 1. If you have any study strategies, high-yield facts with mnemonics, or book reviews for the next edition, please use the forms included to submit your contributions. (*See* How to Contribute, page xv.) Any student or faculty member who submits material subsequently used in the next edition of *First Aid for the USMLE Step 1* will receive personal acknowledgment in the next edition and one $10 coupon per complete entry, good toward the future purchase of any Appleton & Lange medical book.

Good luck in your studies!!

Acknowledgments

This has been a collaborative project from the start. We gratefully acknowledge the thoughtful comments, corrections, and advice of the numerous medical students and faculty who have supported the authors in the development of *First Aid for the USMLE Step 1*.

We were inspired by two established "student-to-student" guides: Macklis, *Introduction to Clinical Medicine, A Student-to-Student Guide* (Little, Brown), and Betcher, *A Student-to-Student Guide to Medical School: Study Strategies, Mnemonics, Personal Growth* (Little, Brown). An impressive example of what a comprehensive review book can become is Dähnert, *Radiology Review Manual* (Williams and Wilkins).

We acknowledge Dr. Donald Melnick (NBME) and Dr. Peter Ralston (Chairman, USMLE Step 1 Committee) for reviewing the exam preparation guide section of the 1992 and 1996 editions respectively. Thanks to Jeanette Jackson and Beth Sullivan for their contributions to the Section I Supplement. For reviewing the anatomy section, we thank Dr. Gerry Cunha, Dr. Hugh "Pat" Patterson, Dr. Peter Ralston and Dr. Steven Rosen from the UCSF Department of Anatomy. For helping us obtain information concerning review books, we thank Joe Libs (Milberry Union Bookstore, UCSF), Sam Morris (Discount Medical Books, San Francisco), Margaret Dawson (Reiter's Scientific & Professional Books, Washington, DC), and Lisa Holster (UCLA Health Sciences Bookstore). Thanks to Noam Maitless for the original book design, Evenson Design Group for interior design revisions, and Design Group Cook for the cover design.

For support and encouragement throughout the process, we are grateful to Karen Bagatelos, Martina Kreidl, Dr. Sana Khan, Dr. Steve McPhee, Dr. Barbara Gastel, Dr. Lawrence Tierney, Ray Moloney (Paper Book Press), Jonathan Kirsch, Esq., Konrad Fernandez, Jean Williams, Michael Lowe, and the UCSF Office of Medical Student Affairs.

Thanks to our publisher, Appleton & Lange, for offering a coupon for each new contribution used in future editions of this book, and for the valuable assistance of their staff. For enthusiasm, support, and commitment for this ongoing and ever challenging project, thanks to our editors, John Dolan and Marinita Timban.

For submitting contributions to the 1996 edition we thank Peter Abdel-Sayed, Matthew Abel, Kenneth Adams, Neagoe Adriana, Suneet Agarwal, Margaret Amateau, Desh Anand, Ritu Anand, Rebecca Archer, Maryam Azizi, Tuvana Bain, Ali Bazzi, Norman Beauchamp, Steve Behr, Heidi Bertram, Rachel Bittker, Michael Bobo, Christina Borroum, J. Breau, Lester Brown, John Cai, Yan Cao, Jaishree Capoor, Mike Carley, Marie Carrier, Corey Casper, Natalie Chantfield, Lisa Christopher, Stephen Cico, Jane Cleary, Bruce Clemons, Orion Colfer, Heena Contractor, Diego Covarrubias, Richard Covey, Angela Crone, Mary Chimura, Chris Chow, Lara Danziger, Erik Davydov, Charley Della Santina, Carl DeMars, Anita Demas, Mark Detherage, Salena Dhillon, Jessie Dill, Jason Dilly, Mike Dixon, Theresa Domers, Amol Doshi, Valery Dronsky, Robert Dudley, Susan Dunn, William Dupon, Stephanie Evans, Linda Lynn Fagan, Elhan Farahabadi, Jessica Feinman, Michelle Fink, Carmel Anne Flores, Michael Fogli, Chris Fox, Deborah Fuchs, Shawn Fultz, Roger Gajraj, Ariel Gildengers, Marina Gorenshteyn, J. M. Grohdahl, Gregory Guldner, Bobby Gupta, Kristina Gutierrez, Derek Haas, Melanie Hartman, Wesley Heartfield, Kim Hiatt, Carole Ho, Letrinh Hoang, Hoch, Heidi Hoffman, Juliet Howard, Tamara Hughes, Hamid Hussain, Darrell Hutson, Charles Jaffe, Alex Janusz, Clark Jean, Lisa Jias, Timothy Jones, Satheesh Kathula, Leon Katz, Jarrod Kaufman, Carla Kazazian, Stephen Kellam, Naiyar Khayyam, Brian Kim, Miriam Klaiman, Edson Knapp, Zee Kogen, Christopher Konalski, Bryan Krol, Wendy Kuohung, Mikyung Kwah, Scott Landry, Robert Latkany, Monique Lawrence, Chang Lee, Steven Lee, John Leisey, Kenneth Levey, Judith Lin, Xiang Lin, Hong Liu, Keri Livingstone, Amy Lockhert, Irene Loe, Sonia Lott, Brian Lucas, Julie MacRae, Arshad Majid, Karen Mark, Paul Martinetti, Donald Maxwell, Mallory McClure, Richard McColl, James McIntyre, Aaron Michelfelder, Darryl Miles, Dan Miller, Joy

Mockbee, Vino Mody, Anbin Mu, T. Naassana, Lori Nizel, Mel Nutter, Rose Obinyan, Jason Pachman, Clara Paik, Clara Palma, Uptal Patel, S. Prakash, Jinha Park, Scott Parkhill, Andrea Pass, Delia Patroi, Marcelo Perez-Montes, Tina Pham, Amy Potter, Paul Quick, Ishrat Rafi, Heidi Rand, Dana Rausch, Kenneth Reed, John Reese, Mark Richman, Jeff Riggio, Joy Rodriguez, Eric Rogoff, Walter Rush, Jeff Ryan, Leon Sanchez, Babak Sarani, Neville Sarkari, Jeffrey Scott, John Scott, Pamela Schutzer, Debby Schwartz, Prerak Shah, Shaji Matthew, Xiaochu Shangguan, Andrew Shapiro, Shaz Siddiqi, Mark Silverberg, Sadhish Siva, Brian Sloan, Brian Smoley, Joy Snyder, Robert Somer, Dan Spevack, Ken Stringer, Lori Summers, Jonathan Svahn, David Tan, Jeff Taylor, Mark Taylor, Vasuki Thangamuthu, Rosy Thind, Bob Titleman, Cathy Tong, Louis Tran, Marcus Trione, John Tsai, Maria Tsangariaov, Daniel Vasiliu-Rab, Phi Vophi, Hui Wang, Antoinette Wassel, Britt Wells, Jule West, Sarah Whang, Julie White, Veronica Williams, Ben Winkes, Kerry Wong, S. Woolsey, Francis Yu and Yuriy Zhukovskiy among others. We apologize if any names have been omitted or misspelled.

For submitting surveys we thank Carla Aamodt, Ty Abel, Theresa Albright, Seth Alpert, Stephanie Anderson, Robert Angert, Deborah Arce, Jessie Backer, Rahil Bandukwala, Angela Basham, Jonathan Bellman, Eventure Bernardino, Mark Bernas, David Bowne, Patricia Burgess, John Burke, Michele Campisi, Steve Cannon, Alisa Carlton, Jennifer Cavitt, Jill Chrispens, Eugene Chu, Brett Cohen, John Cosmi, Tom Cox, Todd Craig, Caren Crane, Heather Crowley, Carrie Cwiak, Michael Dahl, Kim Dehn, Anita Demas, Matt Dickson, Christine Dignan, Nora Dobos, Lee Du, Karin Dydell, Michael Eis, Craig Endo, Kalpana Engineer, Adam Falik, Afshin Farzadmehr, Shirin Farzadmehr, Steven Feigenberg, Michael Flais, D. Fuchs, Deborah Garretts, Janette Gaw, T. Geonzon, Cynthia Gepport, Alberto Ginzo, Justin Graham, Rodelio Guintu, Jay Han, Dennis Harden, Howard Harris, Katherine Hemela, William Henry, Patrick Hinfey, Quynh-Mai Hoang, Josephine Huang, Heidi Huser, Rob Hwong, Beth Johnson, Makroughi Kademian, Andrew Kayser, Teresa Kellogg, Julie Kim, Sara Kim, Lee Kiser, Frank Klanduch, Jennifer Knaak, Joseph Kueter, Eda Kwak, Sandy Lai, Sonia Lee, Inger Leria, Shawn LeTarte, Nikki Levin, Hong Li, Karen Libsch, Joe Liddle, Jerry Limb, Tammy Lin, Tingi Lu, Sarah Lulloff, John Ma, Jules Madrigal-Dersch, Eric Mai, Swarna Manian, Andrea Marcus, Carlos Martinez, Karen Mecklenburg, Yun Miao, Erik Mont, Sanjai Nagendra, Brian Nelson, Julie Neville, Kent New, Malinda Newcombe, Patricia Newland, Jelena Nikolic, Angela Nishio, Mary Norman, Tommy Oei, Brett Ohlfs, Natalie Ong, Catherine Olson, Tom Ormiston, Will Ostdiek, Namrata Patil, Ronjon Paul, Vicente Peralta, Mike Pham, Christopher Pierson, Sapan Polepalle, Jerome Pomear, A. Puskar, Gautham Reddy, Jonathan Reitman, Jack Resneck, Jr., Christopher Ricci, Brian Romias, Lorca Rossman, Richard Roston, Julie Roth, William Ruth, Nathalie Saget, Anita Sahu, Michael Schatzman, Zoey Schorr, Shoshana Schwartz, Jennifer Sellakumar, Sushma Shail, Paige Sharp, Alice Shih, Jennifer Smith, Arthur Sorrell, Jane Speaker, J. Staples, Cedric Strange, Bill Stratbucker, Stacy Stratmann, Arro Sullivan, Shiaochi Sun, Saumya Sutaria, Jon Swerdloff, Jesse Tan, Roland Tang, T. Tchernikova-Ramey, Beverly Tong, Yolanda Troublefield, David Uvrate, Carin Van Gelder, David Vo, Paul Wallace, Jim Wang, Rhonda Weiss, John White, III, Jason Wittmer, Walt Wojnar, Carrie Wong, Sandra Wong, Emily Wu, Kesheng Wu, Ron Wurth, Sophia Yen and Antonia Zazueta among others. Again, we apologize if any names have been omitted or misspelled.

Finally, thanks to Ted Hon, one of the founding authors of this book, for his vision in developing this guide on the computer. Eddie Chu and Jeffrey Hansen were also among the founding authors of this book. For major contributions to previous editions, we thank Matthew Voorsanger, John Bethea, Jr., Ketan Kapadia, Lisa Backus, Yi Chieh Shiuey, Shin Kim, Robert Hosseini, Kassem Kahlil, Dax Swanson, Kathleen Liu, Kieu Nguyen, Hatem Abou-Sayed, Shaun Anand, Radhika Sekhri-Breaden, Stephen Gomperts, Sana Khan, and Thao Pham.

Los Angeles   Vikas Bhushan
San Francisco   Tao Le
Miami   Chirag Amin

How to Contribute

This version of *First Aid for the USMLE Step 1* incorporates hundreds of contributions and changes suggested by faculty and student reviewers. We invite you to participate in this process.

Please send us your suggestions for:

- New facts, mnemonics, diagrams, or strategies
- High-yield topics that may reappear on future Step 1 exams
- Personal ratings and comments on review books that you have examined

For each entry incorporated into the next edition, you will receive one $10 coupon per entry good toward the purchase of any Appleton & Lange medical book, as well as personal acknowledgment in the next edition. Diagrams, tables, partial entries, updates, corrections, and study hints are also appreciated, and significant contributions will be compensated at the discretion of the publisher. Also let us know about material in this edition that you feel is low-yield and should be deleted.

The preferred way to submit entries, suggestions, or corrections is via electronic mail, addressed to:

Vbhushan @ aol.com
Taodoc @ aol.com
Chiragamin @ aol.com

For Step 1 updates and corrections, visit our new Internet Website at:

http: //www.s2smed.com

Otherwise, please send entries, neatly written or typed or on disk (Microsoft Word), to: First Aid for the USMLE Step 1, 1442 Lincoln Avenue, Ste. 146, Orange, CA 92665, Attention: Contributions. Please use the contribution and survey forms on the following pages. Each form constitutes an entry. (Attach additional pages as needed.)

Another option is to send in your entire annotated book. We will look through your additions and notes and will send you Appleton & Lange coupons based on the quantity and quality of any additions that we incorporate into the 1997 edition. Books will be returned upon request. Contributions received by July 15, 1996, receive priority consideration for the 1997 edition of *First Aid for the USMLE Step 1.*

Note to Contributors

All entries are subject to editing and reviewing. Please verify all data and spellings carefully. In the event that similar or duplicate entries are received, only the first entry received will be used. Include a reference to a standard textbook to facilitate verification of the fact. Please follow the style, punctuation, and format of this edition if possible.

Contribution Form I

For entries, mnemonics, facts,
strategies, corrections,
diagrams, etc.

Contributor Name: _____

School/Affiliation: _____

Address: _____

_____

Telephone: _____

Topic:

Fact and Description:

Notes, Diagrams, and Mnemonics:

Reference:

Please return by July 15, 1996. You will receive personal acknowledgment and a $10 coupon toward selected Appleton & Lange books for each entry that we use in future editions.

- (fold here) -

Return Address

_____

_____

_____

| Postage required |

Attn: Contributions
First Aid for the USMLE Step 1
1442 Lincoln Avenue, Ste. 146
Orange, CA 92665

- (fold here) -

Contribution Form II

For high-yield topics for
Section II Supplement

Contributor Name: _____

School/Affiliation: _____

Address: _____

_____

Telephone: _____

Please place the subject headings (e.g., Anatomy) on the first line and the high-yield topic on the following two lines.

1. Subject: _____
   Topic: _____
   _____

2. Subject: _____
   Topic: _____
   _____

3. Subject: _____
   Topic: _____
   _____

4. Subject: _____
   Topic: _____
   _____

5. Subject: _____
   Topic: _____
   _____

6. Subject: _____
   Topic: _____
   _____

7. Subject: _____
   Topic: _____
   _____

8. Subject: _____
   Topic: _____
   _____

9. Subject: _____
   Topic: _____
   _____

10. Subject: _____
    Topic: _____
    _____

Please return by July 15, 1996. You will receive personal acknowledgment and a $10 coupon toward selected Appleton & Lange books for each entry that is used in future editions.

(fold here)

Return Address

_____

_____

_____

Postage
required

Attn: Contributions
First Aid for the USMLE Step 1
1442 Lincoln Avenue, Ste. 146
Orange, CA 92665

(fold here)

Contribution Form III

For review book ratings for
Section III

Contributor Name: _____

School/Affiliation: _____

Address: _____

_____

Telephone: _____

We welcome additional comments on review books rated in Section III as well as reviews of texts not rated in Section III. Please fill out each review entry as completely as possible. Please do not leave "Comments" blank. Rate texts using the letter grading scale provided on p. 218, taking into consideration other books on that subject.

1. *Title/Author:* _____

   Publisher/Series: _____   ISBN Number: _____

   Rating: _____   *Comments:* _____

   _____
   _____

2. *Title/Author:* _____

   Publisher/Series: _____   ISBN Number: _____

   Rating: _____   *Comments:* _____

   _____
   _____

3. *Title/Author:* _____

   Publisher/Series: _____   ISBN Number: _____

   Rating: _____   *Comments:* _____

   _____
   _____
   _____

4. *Title/Author:* _____

   Publisher/Series: _____   ISBN Number: _____

   Rating: _____   *Comments:* _____

   _____
   _____

5. *Title/Author:* _____

   Publisher/Series: _____   ISBN Number: _____

   Rating: _____   *Comments:* _____

   _____
   _____

Please return by July 15, 1996. You will receive personal acknowledgment and a $10 coupon toward selected Appleton & Lange books for each entry that is used in future editions.

(fold here)

Return Address

_____

_____

_____

Postage
required

Attn: Contributions
First Aid for the USMLE Step **1**
1442 Lincoln Avenue, Ste. 146
Orange, CA 92665

(fold here)

User Survey

Contributor Name: _____

School/Affiliation: _____

Address: _____

_____

Telephone: _____

What student-to-student advice would you give someone preparing for the USMLE Step 1?

Are you aware of any commercial review courses not listed in Section I: Guide to Efficient Exam Preparation? If yes, which ones? What commercial courses have you been enrolled in, and what were your overall assessments of the courses?

What would you change about the study and test-taking strategies listed in Section I: Guide to Efficient Exam Preparation?

Were there any high-yield facts or topics in Section II that you think were inaccurate or should be deleted? Which ones and why? What would you change or add?

What review books for the USMLE Step 1 are not covered in Section III? Would you change the rating of any of the review books in Section III? If so, which one(s) and why?

How else would you improve *First Aid for the USMLE Step 1?* Any other comments or suggestions? What did you like most about the book?

Please return by July 15, 1996. You will receive personal acknowledgment and a $10 coupon toward selected Appleton & Lange books for material that is used in future editions.

--(fold here)--

Return Address

_____

_____

_____

Postage
required

Attn: Contributions
First Aid for the USMLE Step 1
1442 Lincoln Avenue, Ste. 146
Orange, CA 92665

--(fold here)--

How to Use This Book

Medical students who have used previous editions of this guide have given us feedback on how best to make use of the book.

It is recommended that you begin using this book as early as possible when learning the basic medical sciences. You can use Section III to select first-year course review books and then use those books for review while taking your medical school classes.

Use different parts of the book at different stages in your preparation for the USMLE Step 1. Before you begin to study for the USMLE Step 1, we suggest that you read Section I: Guide to Efficient Exam Preparation and Section III: Database of Science Review Books. **If you are an international medical graduate or an osteopathic medical student,** refer to the Section I supplement for additional advice. Devise a study plan and decide what resources to buy. Scanning Section II will give you an initial idea of the diverse range of topics covered on the USMLE Step 1.

As you study each discipline, **use the corresponding high-yield fact section in *First Aid for the USMLE Step 1* as a way of consolidating the material and testing yourself** to see if you have covered some of the frequently tested items. Work with the book to integrate important facts into your fund of knowledge. Using *First Aid for the USMLE Step 1* as a review can serve as both a self-test of your knowledge and repetition of important facts to learn.

Return to Section II frequently during your preparation and fill your short-term memory with remaining high-yield facts a few days before the USMLE Step 1. The book can serve as a useful way of retaining key associations and high-yield facts fresh in your memory just prior to the examination. Some students choose to skim the book between the two exam days.

Reviewing the book immediately after the exam is probably the best way to **help us improve the book in the next edition.** Decide what was truly high and low yield and **send in the contribution forms or your entire annotated book.**

Guide to Efficient Exam Preparation

INTRODUCTION

Relax.

This section is intended to make your exam preparation easier, not harder. Our goal is to reduce your stress and help you make the most of your study effort by helping you understand more about the United States Medical Licensing Examination, Step 1 (USMLE Step 1). As a medical student, you are undoubtedly familiar with taking standardized examinations and absorbing large amounts of material. However, in confronting the USMLE Step 1, it is easy to become sidetracked and not achieve your goal of studying with maximum effectiveness. Common mistakes that students make when studying for the boards include the following:

- "Stressing out" due to an inadequate understanding of the test
- Not understanding how scoring is performed and what your score means
- Not utilizing the NBME/USMLE's own publications for maximum benefit
- Starting to study too late
- Using inefficient or inappropriate study methods
- Buying the wrong books or buying more than one can ever use
- Buying only one publisher's review series for all subjects
- Buying review books too late and never reading them
- Not utilizing practice examinations for maximum benefit
- Not analyzing and improving one's test-taking strategies
- Getting bogged down by excessively reviewing difficult topics
- Studying material that is almost never tested on the USMLE Step 1
- Failing to master certain high-yield subjects due to overconfidence

In this section, we will offer advice to help you avoid these pitfalls and be more productive in your studies. First, it is important to understand what the examination involves.

USMLE STEP 1—THE BASICS

The purpose of the USMLE Step 1 is to test your understanding and application of important concepts in basic biomedical sciences. [2]

A degree of concern about one's performance on the USMLE Step 1 examination is expected and appropriate. However, medical students all too often become unnecessarily anxious about the examination. It is important to take a moment to understand what it involves. As you become more familiar with the USMLE Step 1, you can translate your anxiety into more efficient preparation.

The USMLE Step 1 is the first of three examinations that you must pass in order to become a licensed physician in the United States.[1] The USMLE is a joint endeavor of the National Board of Medical Examiners (NBME) and the Federation of State Medical Boards (FSMB). In previous years, the examination was strictly organized around seven traditional disciplines: anatomy, behavioral science, biochemistry, microbiology, pathology, pharmacology, and physiology. In June 1991, the NBME began administering the "new" NBME Part I examination. The new examination offered a more integrated, multidisciplinary format and more **clinically** oriented questions.

In 1992, the USMLE replaced both the Federation Licensing Examination (FLEX) and the certifying examinations of the NBME.[3] The USMLE now serves as the **single** examination system for United States medical students and foreign medical graduates seeking medical licensure.

Format

The USMLE Step 1 is a multiple-choice examination administered over a two-day period (Fig. 1). It consists of four booklets, each containing approximately 185 items. On each day of the examination, one booklet is administered in the morning and one is administered in the afternoon. You are allotted three hours to complete each test booklet. A sample answer sheet and the table of normal laboratory values provided within each booklet are shown in the *USMLE Step 1 General Instructions, Content Outline, and Sample Items.*[4]

FIGURE 1. Schematic of the 1995 USMLE Step 1 Administration

	Day 1	Day 2
	Registration	Seating
3 hours in AM	**Book 1** ~185 questions	**Book 3** ~185 questions
	Lunch	Lunch
3 hours in PM	**Book 2** ~185 questions	**Book 4** ~185 questions

---

Test booklets vary in difficulty, so do not become discouraged early in the exam.

Figure 1 should give you a mental image of the exam structure. Note that:

- Booklets vary in overall difficulty. There does not seem to be a pattern of increasing or decreasing difficulty as you proceed through the exam.
- Subject areas vary randomly from question to question. Many questions incorporate multiple basic science and medical concepts.
- The last booklet is printed on high-quality, glossy paper and includes a number of color photographs. In 1995, some students also reported a black-and-white, glossy booklet during the afternoon of the first day.
- The exam is scored if all four booklets are opened.[5] Otherwise, a notation on the USMLE transcript will be made that the examination was incomplete.

Question Types
One-best-answer items are the most commonly used multiple-choice format. They usually consist of a statement or a question followed by a list of three to five options. You are required to select the one best answer among the options. A number of options may be partially correct, in which case you must select the option that best answers the question or completes the statement. A variation of this format uses negative stems such as EXCEPT, LEAST, and NOT.

About half the Step 1 questions begin with a description of a patient.[6]

Clinical vignettes have become increasingly common in the past few administrations of the USMLE Step 1. They consist of a short description of a clinical case or scenario, often including lab values and radiological images, followed by a question or questions in the one-best-answer format described above.

Matching sets consist of a list of approximately 4 to 26 items from which you choose the one best answer that corresponds with the numbered items or questions located below the list. Once again, a number of options may be partially correct, in which case you must select the option that best answers the question or completes the statement.

Student experience from the June 1995 administration indicates that questions in each booklet are organized by type, starting with the one-best-answer items, followed by negatively phrased one-best-answer items, and ending with matching sets. Though the numerical proportions of question types vary with each booklet, students recall that the one-best-answer items constituted approximately 80 to 90% of all questions, while negatively phrased one-best-answer items constituted about 5% and matching sets made up roughly 10% of the questions each (Fig. 2).

Scoring and Failure Rates
Each Step 1 examinee will receive a score report that has the examinee's pass/fail status, two test scores, and a graphical depiction of the examinee's performance by discipline and organ system or subject area (Fig. 3). The actual

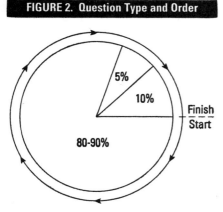

FIGURE 2. Question Type and Order

~80-90% One-best-answer
~5% Negatively phrased one-best-answer
~10% Matching and extended matching

FIGURE 3A. Simulated Score Report–Front Page

Doe, John I.
000 Main St.
Any Town, CA 12345

USMLE ID: 0-123-456-7
Test Date: June 1995

The USMLE is a single examination program for all applicants for medical licensure in the United States; it replaces the Federation Licensing Examination (FLEX) and the certifying examinations of the National Board of Medical Examiners (NBME Parts I, II, and III). The program consists of three Steps designed to assess an examinee's understanding of and ability to apply concepts and principles that are important in health and disease and that constitute the basis of safe and effective patient care. **Step 1** is designed to assess whether an examinee understands and can apply key concepts of the basic biomedical sciences, with an emphasis on principles and mechanisms of health, disease, and modes of therapy. The inclusion of Step 1 in the USMLE sequence is intended to ensure mastery of not only the basic medical sciences undergirding the safe and competent practice of medicine in the present, but also the scientific principles required for maintenance of competence through lifelong learning. Results of the examination are reported to medical licensing authorities in the United States and its territories for use in granting an initial license to practice medicine. The two numeric scores shown below are equivalent; each state or territory may use either score in making licensing decisions. These scores represent your results for the administration of Step 1 on the test date shown above.

PASS	The result is based on the minimum passing score set by USMLE for Step 1. Individual licensing authorities may accept the USMLE-recommended pass/fail result or may establish a different passing score for their own jurisdictions.

200	This score is determined by your overall performance on Step 1. For recent administrations, the mean and standard deviation for first-time examinees from U.S. medical schools are approximately 205 and 20, respectively, with most scores falling between 165 and 245. A score of 176 is set by USMLE to pass Step 1. The standard error of measurement (SEM)* for this scale is four points.

82	This score is also determined by your overall performance on the examination. A score of 82 on this scale is equivalent to a score of 200 on the scale described above. A score of 75 on this scale, which is equivalent to a score of 176 on the scale described above, is set by USMLE to pass Step 1. The SEM* for this scale is one point.

* Your score is influenced by both your general understanding of basic biomedical sciences and the specific set of items selected for this Step 1 examination. The SEM provides an estimate of the range within which your scores might be expected to vary by chance if you were tested repeatedly using similar tests.

FIGURE 4. Score to Percentile Conversion[7]

Three-Digit Score	Anchor Group* (%ile)	June 94** (%ile)
244	99	98
240	98	96
235	97	93
230	94	89
225	89	82
220	83	74
215	76	65
210	67	56
205	57	46
200	48	37
195	38	29
190	29	22
185	21	16
180	15	11
176	**11**	**8**
170	7	5
165	4	4
160	3	2
155	2	2

* Anchor Group June 91 2nd-yr US students
** June 94 US and Canadian 1st-time takers

organ system profiles reported may depend on the statistical characteristics of a given administration of the examination.

For 1995, USMLE provided two overall test scores based on the total number of items answered correctly on the examination. The first score, the three-digit score, was reported as a scaled score, where the mean was 208 and the standard deviation was 20 (Fig. 5). These values were based on the performance of the June 1991 USMLE Step 1 examinee group. This means that a score of 208

FIGURE 3B. Simulated Score Report—Back Page

INFORMATION PROVIDED FOR EXAMINEE USE ONLY

The Performance Profile below is provided solely for the benefit of the examinee.
The USMLE will not provide or verify the Performance Profile for any other person, organization,
or agency.

USMLE STEP 1 PERFORMANCE PROFILE

	Lower Performance	Borderline Performance	Higher Performance
Behavioral Sciences			xxxxxxxxxxx
Biochemistry			xxxxxxxxx
Cardiovascular System			xxxxxxxxxxxxx
Gastrointestinal System			xxxxxxxxxxxxx
General Principles of Health & Disease			xxxxxxx
Gross Anatomy & Embryology		xxxxxxxxxxxxx	
Hematopoietic & Lymphoreticular Systems			xxxxxxxxxxxxxxx
Histology & Cell Biology		xxxxxxxxxxxxx	
Microbiology & Immunology			xxxxxxxxx
Musculoskeletal, Skin & Connective Tissue			xxxxxxxxxxxxxxx
Nervous System/Special Senses		xxxxxxxxx	
Pathology			xxxx*
Pharmacology			xxxxxxx
Physiology		xxxxxxx	
Renal/Urinary Systems		xxxxxxxxxxxx	
Reproductive & Endocrine Systems		xxxxxxxxxxx	
Respiratory System			xxxxxxxxxx*

The above Performance Profile is provided to aid in self-assessment. The shaded area defines a borderline level of performance for each content area; borderline performance is comparable to a HIGH FAIL/LOW PASS on the total test.

Performance bands indicate areas of relative strength and weakness. Some bands are wider than others. The width of a performance band reflects the precision of measurement; narrower bands indicate greater precision. The band width for a given content area is the same for all examinees. An asterisk indicates that your performance band extends beyond the displayed portion of the scale.

Additional information concerning the topics covered in each content area can be found in the *USMLE Step 1 General Instructions, Content Description, and Sample Items.*

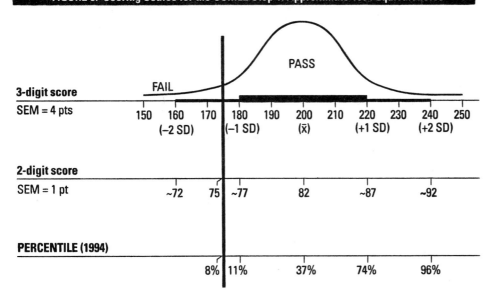

FIGURE 5. Scoring Scales for the USMLE Step 1: Approximate 1994 Equivalencies

roughly corresponded to the 50th percentile, while a score of 225 roughly corresponded to the 85th percentile.[8] The June 1995 USMLE score report for students did not include any percentile score equivalents. 1994 percentile performance norms were provided to medical schools and have been summarized in Figure 4. The second score scale, the two-digit score, defines 75 as the minimum passing score (equivalent to a score of 176 on the first scale). A score of 82 is equivalent to a score of 200 on the first score scale. To avoid confusion, we will refer to scores using the three-digit scale with a current mean of 208 and a standard deviation of 20.

The mean Step 1 score for US medical students rose from 200 in 1991 to 208 in 1995.

A score of 176 or higher is required to pass Step 1. The pass/fail standard for Step 1 is predominantly "content-based." The passing mark was determined by reviewing test items and defining a mastery level of performance.[9] In 1994, 92% of all first-time test takers passed the June administration of the USMLE Step 1 (Fig. 6). With 92% of all first-time test takers also passing the June 1995 USMLE Step 1, the failure rate appears to have stabilized (Fig. 7). However, the mean score for Step 1 continues to rise. The mean score for first-time test takers in the United States was 208 for the June 1995 Step 1 exam.

It is estimated that passing Step 1 will correspond to answering between 55 and 65% of the questions correctly. After extensive review by the USMLE Step 1 committee in 1995, the pass/fail standard of 176 was unchanged and will likely remain so until the next substantive reevaluation in 1998.

Each three-digit scale point is equivalent to about three questions answered correctly.[10]

According to the USMLE, medical schools receive a listing of total scores and pass/fail results plus group summaries by discipline and organ systems. Students can withhold their scores from their medical school if they wish. Official

FIGURE 6. Passing Rates for 1994 USMLE Step 1[11]						
NBME-Registered Examinees	**June 1994**		**September 1994**		**Total 1994**	
First-Time Takers	15,580	92%	1,415	78%	16,995	91%
Repeaters	851	49%	1,396	58%	2,247	54%
NBME Total	**16,431**	**90%**	**2,811**	**68%**	**19,242**	**86%**
ECFMG*-Registered Examinees						
First-Time Takers	7,273	49%	10,176	52%	17,449	51%
Repeaters	4,160	31%	5,165	31%	9,325	31%
ECFMG Total	**11,433**	**42%**	**15,341**	**45%**	**26,774**	**44%**

*Educational Commission for Foreign Medical Graduates.

USMLE transcripts, which can be sent on request to residency programs, will include only total scores, not performance profiles.

The preceding information is based on students' experience with the June 1994 and June 1995 administrations of the USMLE Step 1 and information published by the NBME (refer to the NBME publications listed in the following section). The format and the scoring of the examination are subject to change, and it is best to consult the latest NBME publications and your medical school for the most current and accurate information regarding the examination.

NBME/USMLE Publications

We strongly encourage students to utilize the free materials provided by the testing agencies (see page 25), to study in detail the following NBME publications, and to retain them for future reference:

FIGURE 7. Trends in Performance on USMLE Step 1[12]

	Percent Failing (< 176)	Percent > 225
1991	11	10
1992	9	11
1993	7	14
1994	8	11
1995	8	15

(NBME-registered first-time test takers only)

- *USMLE Step 1 General Instructions, Content Outline, and Sample Items* (information given free to all examinees)
- *USMLE Bulletin of Information* (information given free to all examinees)
- *Retired NBME Basic Medical Sciences (Part I) Test Items* (out of print)
- *Self-Test in the Part I Basic Medical Sciences* (out of print)

The *USMLE Step 1 General Instructions, Content Outline, and Sample Items* booklet contains approximately 120 questions that are identical in format and similar in content to the questions on the actual USMLE Step 1. This practice test is one of the best methods for assessing your boards test-taking skills. However, it does not contain enough questions to simulate the full length of the examination, and its content is a very limited sample of the possible basic science material covered. The extremely detailed 25-page Step I Content Outline provided by the USMLE has not proved useful for students studying for the exam. The USMLE even states that "the content outline is not intended as a guide for curriculum development or as a study guide."[13] We concur with this assessment.

The *USMLE Bulletin of Information* booklet accompanies application materials for the USMLE. This publication has detailed procedural and policy information regarding the USMLE, including descriptions of all three Steps, scoring of the exams, reporting of scores to medical schools and residency programs, procedures for score rechecks and other inquiries, policies for irregular behavior, and test dates.

The *Retired NBME Basic Medical Sciences (Part I) Test Items* contains nearly 1000 "retired" questions, the content of which frequently reappears on the new USMLE Step 1. This publication allows you to assess your performance on each topic and identify areas of weakness. The retired test items include old NBME Part I questions of the K (multiple true/false) and C (A/B/both/neither) variety, neither of which appears on the USMLE Step 1. Although these question types will not be found on the current version of the boards, the **content** of these questions is still relevant.

Another NBME publication very useful to medical students is the *Self-Test in the Part I Basic Medical Sciences,* with 630 questions drawn from the old NBME Part I item pool. It can be used in the same way as the *Retired NBME Basic Sciences (Part I) Test Items.* There is some overlap in content between the two publications. Unfortunately, these question booklets are **no longer available from the NBME.** Some medical schools, however, still have old copies of these booklets available for their students. Another source would be third- and fourth-year students who have saved their copies.

The original questions are becoming more difficult to find every year. However, answer summaries to all 1623 questions in the *Retired* and *Self-Test* booklets are available as an independent publication titled *Underground Guide to Retired and Self-Test Questions.* This publication is available at (800) 247-6553 (see page 221 for more information).

The most productive way to use these study aids is to take the practice examinations and to identify carefully the questions that were missed or that were answered correctly by guessing. Students often find that many missed questions originate from a limited number of seemingly trivial topics (e.g., congenital diseases involving sphingolipid synthesis). It is worthwhile to study these subjects thoroughly, since student experience has shown that the topics covered in these retired questions (trivial or not) **remain predictors** of many topics tested on the new USMLE Step 1.

Though the NBME Self-Test and Retired Test Items are both out of print, they remain a good source of practice questions for the USMLE Step 1.

In summary, these old NBME publications contain many questions that still approximate the style and content of questions appearing on recent USMLE Step 1 examinations. Moreover, some of these questions remain superior to those found in most commercial review books currently on the market. Thus, we suggest that you study all questions available from the NBME before taking the examination. Use a portion of the questions early to assess your strengths and weaknesses; save some questions for a few weeks before the exam to evaluate your progress.

DEFINING YOUR GOALS

It is useful to define your own personal performance goals when approaching the USMLE Step 1. Your style and intensity of preparation can then be matched to your goals. Your goals may depend on your school's requirements, your specialty choice, your grades to date, and/or your personal assessment of test importance.

Just Pass the Exam

As mentioned earlier, the USMLE Step 1 is the first of three standardized examinations that you must pass to become a licensed physician in the United States. For many medical schools, passing the USMLE Step 1 is also required before you can continue with your clinical training. The NBME, however, feels that medical schools should not use Step 1 as the sole determinant of being advanced to the third year.[14] If you are headed for a "noncompetitive" residency program and you have consulted advisers and fourth-year medical students in your area of interest, you may feel comfortable with this approach.

Beat the Mean

Although the NBME warns against the misuse of examination scores to evaluate student qualifications for residency positions, some residency program directors continue to use Step 1 scores to screen applicants.[15] Thus, many students feel it is important to score higher than the national average.

Fourth-year medical students will have the best feel for how Step 1 scores factor into residency applications.

Internship and residency programs vary greatly in their requests for scores. Some simply request your pass/fail status, whereas others request your total score. Some programs have been known to request a photocopy of your score report to determine how well you performed on the individual sections; however, this is unusual. It is unclear how the continuing changes in the USMLE Step 1 examination and score reporting will affect the application process for residency programs. The best sources of bottom-line information are fourth-year medical students who have recently completed the residency application process.

First Aid for the USMLE Step 1 has conducted a small informal post-match survey of fourth-year medical students at several US medical schools regarding

FIGURE 8. Informal Post-Match Survey: Step 1 Goals*		
Just Pass	**Beat the Mean**	**Ace the Exam**
Pediatrics	Emergency Medicine	Dermatology
Family Practice	OB/Gyn	ENT
Internal Medicine	Radiology	Orthopedics
Anesthesiology	General Surgery	Ophthalmology
Psychiatry		

* Based on the results of 110 respondents to an informal survey distributed to US fourth-year medical students at UCSF, UCLA, the University of Louisville, and the University of Miami.

the use of Step 1 scores. Preliminary results are summarized in Figure 8. Use this information only as a rough guide for goal setting.

Some medical students may wish to "beat the mean" for their own personal satisfaction. For these students, there may be a psychological advantage to scoring above the national average.

Ace the Exam

Certain highly competitive residency programs, such as those in ophthalmology and orthopedic surgery, have acknowledged the use of Step 1 scores in their selection process. In such residency programs greater emphasis may be placed on attaining a high score, so students who wish to enter these programs may want to consider aiming for a very high score on the USMLE Step 1. However, use of the USMLE scores for residency selection has been criticized because neither Step 1 nor Step 2 was designed for this purpose.[16] Additionally, only a subset of the basic science facts and concepts that are tested is important to functioning well on the wards. Alternatively, some students may wish to score well in order to feel a sense of mastery as they complete the basic science years.

Some competitive residency programs use Step 1 scores in their selection process.

TIMELINE FOR STUDY

Make a Schedule

After you have defined your goals, map out a study schedule consistent with your objectives, your vacation time, and the difficulty of your ongoing course-work (Fig. 9). Determine whether you want to spread out your study time or concentrate it into 14-hour study days in the final weeks. Also, factor in your own history in preparing for standardized examinations (e.g., SAT, MCAT), but remember that the USMLE Step 1 is longer and covers far more material than other tests you may have taken.

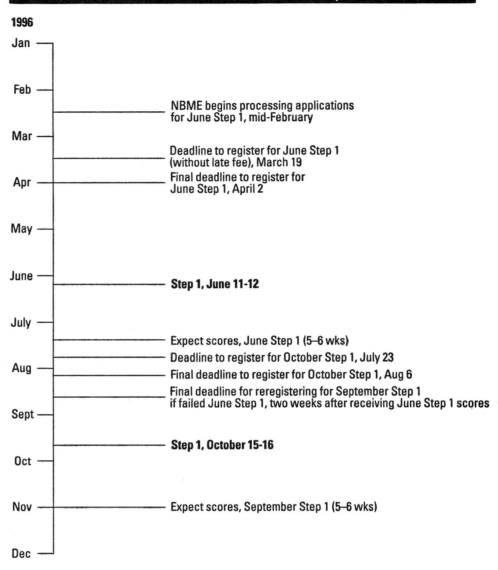

FIGURE 9. Timeline for 1996 USMLE Step 1

1996

- NBME begins processing applications for June Step 1, mid-February
- Deadline to register for June Step 1 (without late fee), March 19
- Final deadline to register for June Step 1, April 2
- **Step 1, June 11-12**
- Expect scores, June Step 1 (5–6 wks)
- Deadline to register for October Step 1, July 23
- Final deadline to register for October Step 1, Aug 6
- Final deadline for reregistering for September Step 1 if failed June Step 1, two weeks after receiving June Step 1 scores
- **Step 1, October 15-16**
- Expect scores, September Step 1 (5–6 wks)

"Crammable" subjects should be covered later and less "crammable" subjects earlier.

Another important consideration is when you will study each subject. Some subjects lend themselves to cramming, whereas others demand a substantial long-term commitment. The "crammable" subjects for Step 1 are those for which concise yet relatively complete review books are available. The three subjects with the most complete and concise review books are microbiology, pharmacology, and biochemistry. (See Section III for highly rated review and sample examination books.) Thus, these three subjects could be covered toward the end of your schedule, whereas other subjects (anatomy, physiology, and pathology) require a longer time commitment and could be studied earlier. Practically speaking, spending a given amount of time on a crammable or high-yield subject (particularly in the waning days before the test) generally produces more correct answers on the examination than spending the same amount of time on a low-yield subject. Student opinion indicates that knowing the crammable subjects extremely well will probably result in a higher overall score than knowing all the subjects moderately well.

If you are having difficulty deciding when to start your test preparation, you may find the reverse-calendar approach helpful. Start with the day of the test and plan backward, setting deadlines for objectives to be met. Where the planning ends on your calendar defines a possible starting point.

Make your schedule realistic, with achievable goals. Many students make the mistake of studying at a level of detail that requires too much time for a comprehensive review—reading *Gray's Anatomy* in a couple of days is not a realistic goal! Revise your schedule regularly based on your actual progress. Be careful not to lose focus. Beware of feelings of inadequacy when comparing study schedules and progress with your peers. Don't set yourself up for frustration.

You will need time for uninterrupted and focused study. Plan your personal affairs to minimize crisis situations near the date of the test. For example, don't get pregnant nine months before the test. Allot an adequate number of breaks in your study schedule to avoid burnout. Maintain a healthy lifestyle, with proper diet and exercise. Getting sick before or during the test will not help your cause.

Year(s) Prior

USMLE asserts that the best preparation for the USMLE Step 1 is "broadly based learning that establishes a strong general foundation of understanding of concepts and principles in basic sciences."[17] We agree. Though you may be tempted to rely solely on "cramming" in the weeks and months before the test to pass, you should not have to. The knowledge gained during your first two years of medical school and even during your undergraduate years provides the groundwork on which to base your test preparation. The majority of your boards preparation will involve resurrecting dormant information stored away during the basic science years. We recommend that you buy highly rated review books early in your first year of medical school and use them as you study throughout the two years. When Step 1 comes along, the books will be more familiar and will be personalized to the way in which you learn.

Buy review books early and use while studying for courses.

Talk to third- and fourth-year medical students to familiarize yourself with strengths and weaknesses in your school's curriculum. Identify subject areas in which you excel or with which you have difficulty. Content typically learned in the second year receives more coverage on Step 1 than do first-year topics due to the emphasis placed on integration of basic science information across many courses.[18] Be aware of your school's testing format and determine whether or not you have adequate exposure to multiple-choice or matching questions.

Month(s) Prior

Review test dates and the application procedure. In 1996, the dates of the USMLE Step 1 are June 11–12 and October 15–16 (Fig. 10).

Simulate the USMLE Step 1 under "real" conditions before beginning your studies.

Before you begin to study earnestly, simulate the USMLE Step 1 under "real" conditions to pinpoint strengths and weaknesses in knowledge and test-taking skills. Be sure that you are well informed about the examination and have planned your strategy for studying. Consider what study methods you will use, the study materials you will need, and how you will obtain your materials. Some review books may not be available at your local bookstore, and you may have to order ahead of time to get copies (see list of publisher contacts at the end of Section III). Plan ahead. Get advice from third- and fourth-year medical students who have recently taken the USMLE Step 1. There might be strengths and weaknesses in your school's curriculum that you should take into account in deciding where to focus your efforts. Plan how you might be able to pool resources. You might choose to share books, notes, and study hints with classmates. That is how this book began.

Three Weeks Prior

Two to four weeks before the examination is a good time to resimulate the USMLE Step 1. You may want to do this earlier, depending on the progress of your review, but don't do it later, when there will be little time to remedy defects in your knowledge or test-taking skills. Make use of remaining good-quality sample USMLE test questions and try to simulate the test conditions so that you gain a fair assessment of your test performance.

One Week Prior

Make sure you have your admission ticket and items necessary for the day of the examination, including five or six #2 pencils, a non-beeping digital timer, and non-smudge erasers. Review the site location and test time. Work out how

FIGURE 10. Test Dates for USMLE Step 1, Step 2, and Step 3*

	Step 1	Step 2	Step 3
1996	June 11–12 October 15–16	March 5–6 August 27–28	May 14–15 December 3–4
1997	June 10–11 October 14–15	March 4–5 August 26–27	May 13–14 December 2–3
1998	June 9–10 October 13–14	March 3–4 August 25–26	May 12–13 December 1–2

* Only 1996 test dates are confirmed.

you will get to the test site and what parking and traffic problems you might encounter. Visit the testing site if possible to get a better idea of the testing conditions. Determine what you will do for lunch. Make sure you have everything you need to ensure that you will be comfortable and alert at the test site (e.g., seat cushions, earplugs, your favorite talismans). If you must travel a long distance to the test site, consider arriving the day before and staying overnight with a friend or at a nearby hotel.

One Day Prior

Relax and rest the night before the test. Double-check your admissions and test-taking materials as well as comfort measures as discussed above so you do not have to deal with such details the morning of the exam. Do not study any new material. If you feel compelled to study, then quickly review short-term-memory material (e.g., Section II: Database of High-Yield Facts) before going to sleep (the brain does a lot of information processing at night). However, do not quiz yourself, as you may risk becoming flustered and confused. Don't panic and don't underestimate your ability. Many students report difficulty sleeping the night prior to the exam. Do whatever it takes to ensure a good night's sleep (e.g., massage, exercise, warm milk).

Ensure that you will be comfortable and alert.

Morning of the Exam

Wake up at your regular time and eat a normal breakfast. Drink coffee, tea, or soda in moderation, or you may end up wasting exam time on bathroom breaks. Make sure you have your admission ticket, test-taking materials, and comfort measures as discussed above. Wear loose, comfortable clothing. Plan for a variable temperature in the testing center. Remember that you will arrive early in the morning, when it may be cool, and you will not leave until late in the afternoon, when it may be warmer. Arrive at the test site a few minutes before the time designated on the admission ticket; do not come too early, as this may increase anxiety. Seating will be assigned, but ask to be reseated if necessary. You need to be seated in an area that will allow you to remain comfortable and concentrate. Some students find that sitting in the very front or the very back of the room is the least distracting. Listen to your proctors regarding any changes in instructions or testing procedures specific to your test site.

No notes, books, calculators, pagers, recording devices, or alarm timers are allowed. If you must leave, you will be escorted and will not receive extra time.

Remember that it is natural (and even beneficial) to be a little nervous. Focus on being mentally clear and alert. Avoid panic. When asked to begin each booklet, catch your breath, read the directions carefully, rapidly skim the entire booklet, and then begin. Remember your time budget. If time and the testing center permit, take breaks to stretch and relax.

The lunch break is an excellent opportunity to recover, relax, and reorganize your thoughts. Some students utilize the break to discuss questions with

Certain "theme" topics tend to recur throughout the exam and across both days.

classmates or look up information. Also, some students recommend reviewing theme topics during lunch and between days one and two. However, do what feels comfortable. If you decide to review the morning session, do not dwell on perceived mistakes. Remain focused and briefly review topics that you feel are likely to reappear

Between the First and Second Days

Relax. You will need the rest to avoid fatigue on the second day. Maintain a positive attitude and do not be discouraged. If you feel absolutely compelled, you can lightly review short-term memory material or "theme" topics heavily tested on the first day. Do a quick analysis of your test-taking technique and how you might modify it for the second day. Assess if your pace of answering questions was too slow, too fast, or just right. Again, do whatever it takes to ensure a good night's sleep.

After the Test

Have fun and relax regardless of the outcome. Taking the test is an achievement in itself. Enjoy the free time you have before your clerkships. Once you have sufficiently recovered from the test (or from partying), we invite you to send us your feedback, corrections, and suggestions for entries, facts, mnemonics, strategies, book ratings, etc. (*See* How to Contribute, p. xv.) Sharing your experience will benefit fellow medical students and foreign medical graduates.

IF YOU THINK YOU FAILED

After the test, many examinees feel that they have failed, and most are at least unsure of their pass/fail status. There are several sensible steps you can take to plan for the future if you do not achieve a passing score. First, save and organize all your study materials, including review books, practice tests, and notes. If you studied from borrowed materials, make sure that you have immediate access to them. Review your school's policy regarding requirements for graduation and promotion to the third year. About half of the medical schools accredited by the Liaison Committee on Medical Education require passing Step 1 for promotion to the third year, and two-thirds require passing Step 1 as a requirement for graduation.[19] Even if passing Step 1 is not necessary for promotion to the third year, it is probably best to retake the exam at the next available administration. Weigh your options carefully. Finally, familiarize yourself with reapplication procedures for Step 1, including application deadlines and upcoming test dates.

USMLE Step 1 results usually arrive in the mail about six weeks after the test administration. If you do not achieve a passing score on the June administration of Step 1, then you have about eight weeks to prepare for the September Step 1. The deadline for the September administration is generally extended two weeks past the June Step 1 score mailings for examinees who fail and wish to repeat the exam.[20] If you believe that your scores were incorrectly determined, you may request that your answer sheets be rechecked by hand. The resulting scores will be honored. The request must be submitted in writing with a fee to the test administration entity that registered you for the Step 1. The performance profiles on the back of the USMLE Step 1 score report provide valuable feedback concerning your relative strengths and weaknesses (Fig. 3B). Study the performance profiles closely. Then, set up a study timeline to repair defects in knowledge as well as to maintain and improve what you already know. (*See* Timeline for Study, p. 11.) Do not neglect high-yield subjects. Finally, it is absolutely normal to feel somewhat anxious about retaking the test. But if anxiety becomes a problem, seek appropriate counseling.

Sixty percent of the NBME-registered first-time takers who failed the June 1994 Step 1 repeated the exam in September. The overall pass rate for that group in September was 64%. However, pass rates varied widely depending on previous performance on the June 1994 administration (Fig. 11).

Though NBME allows an unlimited number of attempts to pass the Step 1, both the NBME and the FSMB recommend that licensing authorities allow a minimum of three and a maximum of six attempts for each Step examination.[22] Again, review your school's policy regarding retakes.

FIGURE 11. Pass Rates for USMLE Step 1 Repeaters 1994[21]

Score in June	Percent Passing in September
173–175	88%
170–172	89%
165–169	72%
160–164	49%
150–159	26%
<150	6%
Overall	**64%**

STUDY METHODS

It is important to have a set of study methods for preparing for the USMLE Step 1. There is too much material to study by random reading and memorization. Experiment with different ways of studying. You don't know how effective something might be until you try it. This is best done months before the test in order to determine what works and what you enjoy. Possible study options include:

- Studying review material in groups
- Creating personal mnemonics, diagrams, and tables
- Taking practice tests alone or in groups
- Attending faculty review sessions
- Making or sharing flashcards
- Reviewing old syllabi and notes
- Making cassette tapes of review material to study during commuting time
- Playing Trivial Pursuit–style games with facts and questions

■ Getting away from home for an extended period to avoid distractions and to immerse oneself in studying

Study Groups

A good study group has many advantages. It can relieve stress, organize your time, and allow people with different strengths to exchange information. Study groups also allow you to pool resources and spend less money on review books and sample tests.

There are, however, potential problems with study groups. It is difficult to study with people who have different goals and study paces. Avoid large, unwieldly groups. Otherwise, studying can be inefficient and time-consuming. Some study groups also tend to socialize more than study.

If you choose not to belong to a study group, it may be a good idea to find a support group or study partner simply to keep pace with and share study ideas. It is good to get different perspectives from other students in evaluating what is and is not important to learn.

Mnemonics and Memorizing

Developing mnemonics takes time and work.

Cramming is a viable way of memorizing short-term information just before a test, but after one or two days you will find that much of that knowledge has dissipated. For that reason, cramming and memorization by repetition ("brute force") are not ideal techniques for long-term memorization of the overwhelming body of information covered by Step 1 in the weeks before the exam. Mnemonics are memory aids that work by linking isolated facts or abstract ideas to acronyms, pictures, patterns, rhymes, and stories—information that the mind tends to store well.[23] The best mnemonics are your own, and developing them takes work. The first step to creating a mnemonic is understanding the information to be memorized. Play around with the information and look for unique features that will help you remember it. In addition, make the mnemonic as colorful, humorous, or outlandish as you can; such mnemonics are the most memorable. In memorizing the mnemonic, engage as many senses as possible by repeating the fact aloud or writing or acting it out. Keep the information fresh by periodically quizzing yourself with flashcards, in study groups, etc. Do not make the common mistake of simply rereading highlighted review material. The material may start to look familiar, but that does not mean you will be able to remember it in another context during the exam.

Quiz yourself periodically. Do not simply reread highlighted material.

Review Sessions

Faculty review sessions can be helpful. Review sessions that are focused at the level of emphasis of the USMLE Step 1 tend to be more helpful than general review sessions. Open "question and answer" sessions tend to be inefficient and not worth the time. Focus on reviews given by faculty who are knowledgeable in the content and testing format of the USMLE Step 1.

Commercial Courses

Commercial preparation courses can be helpful for some students, but they are expensive and require significant time commitment. They are usually effective in organizing study material for students who feel overwhelmed by the volume of material. Note that the multi-week courses may be quite intense and, thus, leave limited time for independent study. Note that some commercial courses are designed for first-time test takers and that others focus on students who are repeating the examination. Some courses focus on foreign medical graduates who must take all three Steps in a limited amount of time. See page 259 for summarized data and excerpted information from several commercial review courses.

STUDY MATERIALS

Quality and Cost Considerations

Although there is a plethora of boards review books on the market, the quality of the material is highly variable. Some common problems:

- Certain review books are too detailed for review in a reasonable amount of time or cover subtopics not emphasized on the exam (e.g., a 400-page histology book).
- Many sample question books were originally written over 10 years ago and have not been updated adequately to reflect the new USMLE Step 1.
- Many sample question books use poorly written questions or contain factual errors.
- Explanations for sample questions range from nonexistent to overly detailed.

Review Books

Most review books are the product of considerable effort by experienced educators. There are many, and you must choose which ones to buy based on their relative merits. Although recommendations from other medical students are useful, many students simply recommend whatever books they used without having compared them to other books on the same subject. Don't waste time with very outdated "hand-me-down" review books. Some students blindly advocate one publisher's series without considering the broad range of quality encountered within most series. Weigh different opinions against each other, read the reviews and ratings in Section III of this guide, and choose review books very carefully. You are investing not only money but also your limited study time. Don't worry about finding the "perfect" book, as many subjects simply don't have one, and different students prefer different styles.

There are two types of review books: those that are stand-alone titles and those that are part of a series. The books in a series generally have the same style, and you must decide if that style is helpful for you. However, a given style is not optimal for every subject. For example, charts and diagrams may be the best approach for physiology and biochemistry, whereas tables and outlines may be the better approach for microbiology.

Find out which books are up to date. Some new editions represent major improvements, whereas others contain only cursory changes. You should take into consideration how a book reflects the format of the USMLE Step 1. Note that some of the books reviewed in Section III were published before the introduction of the new USMLE Step 1. Those books that emphasize obscure facts and minute details tend to be less helpful for the USMLE Step 1, since there are now fewer "picky" questions.

When possible, try to use the same books for medical school exam review and Step 1 review.

Texts, Syllabi, and Notes

Use texts and syllabi with care. Many textbooks are generally too detailed for high-yield boards review and include material that is generally not tested on the USMLE Step 1 (e.g., drug dosages, complex chemical structures). Syllabi often reflect the emphasis of the faculty, which may not correspond to the emphasis of the boards. Old class notes have the advantage of presenting material in the way you learned it but suffer from the same disadvantages as syllabi. When using texts or notes, engage in **active learning** by making tables, diagrams, new mnemonics, and conceptual associations whenever possible. Supplement incomplete or unclear material with reference to other appropriate textbooks. Keep a good medical dictionary at hand to sort out definitions.

Practice Tests

Don't waste your time with outdated or overly difficult questions.

Taking practice tests provides valuable information about strengths and weaknesses in your fund of knowledge and test-taking skills. Some students use practice examinations simply as a means of breaking up the monotony of studying and adding variety to their study schedule. Other students study almost solely from practice tests. There is a wide range of quality in available practice material, and it is easy to become frustrated by low-quality sample questions or questions without explanations. Approach sample examinations critically, and don't waste time with low-quality questions until you have exhausted better sources.

Use practice tests to identify concepts and areas of weaknesses, not just facts that you missed.

After taking a practice test, try to identify concepts and areas of weakness, not just the facts that you missed. Don't panic if you miss a lot of questions on a practice examination. Use the experience to motivate your study and prioritize what areas you need to work on the most.

Use quality practice examinations to improve test-taking skills. Analyze your ability to pace yourself so that you have enough time to complete each test booklet comfortably. Practice examinations are also a good means of training yourself to concentrate for long periods of time. Consider taking practice tests with a friend or in a small group to increase motivation and simulate more accurately the format and schedule of the real examination. Analyze the pattern of your responses to questions and determine if you have made systematic errors in answering questions. Common mistakes are reading too much into the question, second-guessing your initial impression, and misinterpreting the question.

GENERAL STUDY STRATEGIES

The USMLE Step 1 was created according to an integrated outline that organizes basic science material in a multidisciplinary approach. Broad-based knowledge is more important than in prior years, so the old adage, "Just study bugs, drugs, and biochem" is not enough to ensure that you do well on USMLE Step 1. The exam is designed to test basic science material and its application to clinical situations. About half of the questions include clinical situations, although some are very brief.

Despite the change in the organization of the subject matter, the detailed Step 1 content outline provided by the USMLE has not proved useful for students. We feel that it is still best to approach the material along the lines of the seven traditional disciplines. In Section II, we provide suggestions on how to approach the material within each subject. We also list some topics that are often neglected.

Practice questions that include case histories or descriptive vignettes will be helpful in preparing yourself for the clinical slant of the USMLE Step 1. We suggest going through a number of quality practice questions from NBME publications or updated review books to get a feel for what is expected of you, but do not get bogged down in studying case histories. It is not necessary to memorize all normal laboratory values, since they are printed on the insides of both the front and back covers of all test booklets. Approaching the USMLE Step 1 along the lines of the disciplines outlined in Section II (especially the high-yield areas) has proven to be the most productive method of studying among students in our survey.

TEST-TAKING STRATEGIES

Your test performance will be influenced by both your fund of knowledge and your test-taking skills. You can increase your performance by considering each of these factors. Test-taking skills and strategies should be developed and perfected well in advance of the test date so you can concentrate on the test itself. We suggest you try the following strategies to see if they might work for you.

Practice and perfect test-taking skills and strategies well before the test date.

Pacing

You have 180 minutes to complete approximately 185 questions. This works out to 62 questions per hour and about 58 seconds per question. We recommend that you give yourself an average of 55 seconds per question or answer 66 questions per hour. This will allow you to have about 10 minutes at the end of the examination to go over any particularly difficult questions that you may have guessed or skipped. Some students prefer to mark a temporary answer on all skipped questions in case they don't have time to return. You may find that some question types (e.g., extended matching) may require less time to process than others. Dealing with such question types first will prevent you from leaving quickly answerable questions unanswered.

An NBME analysis of previous board examinations revealed that some students left a few items unanswered in the first examination book of the first morning.[24] This indicates that pacing yourself may be especially important when working on the first booklet. Make the necessary pacing adjustments as you work on each booklet. Pacing errors leading to unanswered questions have been known to occur even among very well prepared students.

Dealing with Each Question

There are several established techniques for efficiently approaching multiple-choice questions. See what works for you. All questions can be identified as easy, workable, or impossible. Your goal should be to answer all easy questions, to work out all workable questions in a reasonable amount of time, and to make quick and intelligent guesses on all impossible questions. In general, when you eliminate an incorrect choice on a question, mark it out to avoid rereading it unnecessarily. If you are unsure about a choice, place a question mark by it. When you think you have determined the best answer, circle it and mark your answer sheet accordingly.

Difficult Questions

Do not dwell excessively on questions that you are on the verge of "figuring out." Make your best guess and move on.

Questions on the USMLE Step 1 will require varying amounts of time to answer. Some problem-solving questions will take longer than simple, fact-recall questions. Because of the exam's clinical emphasis, you may find that many of the questions appear workable but take more time than is available. It can be tempting to dwell on these types of questions for an excessive amount of time because you will feel you are on the verge of "figuring it out." Resist this temptation and budget your time. Answer the question with your best guess, make a mark signifying "tentative" on your booklet or answer sheet, and come back to the question after you have completed the rest of the booklet. This will keep you from inadvertently leaving any blank questions in your efforts to beat the clock. Remember to save a few minutes at the end to remove all stray marks from the answer sheet and to make sure that all questions have been answered.

Inevitably, there will be some questions for which you will not have a clue (i.e., impossible questions). Don't be disturbed by these questions. Guess and move on. As a medical student, you are used to scoring well on standardized examinations (otherwise you wouldn't be in medical school), and so the USMLE Step 1 may be your first experience with facing lots of questions to which you don't know the answers. Prepare yourself for this. After narrowing down the answers as best you can, have a plan for guessing so that you don't waste time. Remember that you are not expected to know all the answers.

Another reason for not dwelling too long on any question is that certain questions may be **experimental** or may be **printed incorrectly.** Not all questions are scored. Some questions serve as "embedded pre-test items" that will not count toward your overall score.[25] Students have also noted several printing errors in past USMLE Step 1 examinations. The lesson here is that you should not waste too much time with ambiguous or "flawed" questions. The reason you are having difficulty with the question may lie in the question itself and not with you!

Clinical Vignettes

Though half the questions on the Step 1 feature a clinical slant, do not be intimidated. Most clinical vignettes are simply basic science problems presented in the context of a clinical scenario. Look for the underlying basic science principle or fact when you encounter a clinical vignette. Some students suggest adopting an aggressive approach toward longer vignettes. This would include reading the question first, skimming over the answers, and then working back through the clinical history, laboratory data, and diagnostic studies as needed. Other clinical vignettes can be answered directly without reviewing the preliminary material.

Look for the basic science principle or fact behind the clinical vignette.

Batch Fill-in

Most students mark their answer sheet after answering each question. However, constantly shifting back and forth between the test booklet and the answer sheet can break concentration and impart a small but significant time penalty. Batch fill-in separates the tasks of answering the questions and transcribing the answers. First, clearly mark answers in the margin of the test booklet as you do each question, and then carefully transcribe two pages' worth of answers onto the answer sheet before turning the page. Batch fill-in may improve your concentration by keeping your eyes focused on the booklet and help you develop a good question-answer rhythm. You may want to revert to transcribing answers question by question toward the end of each test session. In addition, some students recommend using a dull pencil to fill in the answer sheet because it may be faster. Batch fill-in does not work for everyone. Do not use batch fill-in unless you have practiced it extensively.

Margin Marking

Feel free to write in the test booklet and circle or underline key phrases. Draw diagrams or make notes concerning specific facts when encountering case histories or descriptive vignettes. Focus on specific "buzzwords" within the clinical histories. If you find it helpful, circle important directions and repeated words in the answers. Many students mark the possible answers as "T," "F," or "?" to work out difficult questions.

Guessing

There is **no penalty** for wrong answers. Thus, no answer sheet should be turned in with unanswered questions. A hunch is probably better than a random guess. If you have to guess, we suggest guessing an answer you recognize over one that is totally unfamiliar. If you have studied the subject and do not recognize a particular answer, then it is more likely a distracter than a correct answer. Remember, however, that distracters are carefully written and edited to appear reasonable to all but the most competent examinees. Unlike many other standardized tests, such as the SAT, questions do not appear to increase in difficulty as you progress through each booklet.

The conventional wisdom regarding "reconsidering" answers is not to change answers that you have already marked unless there is a convincing, logical reason to do so—i.e., go with your first hunch. You can test this strategy for yourself by keeping a running total of the questions on which you seriously considered changing your answer when taking practice exams. Experience will eventually tell you when to trust your first hunches.

Fourth-Quarter Effect (Avoiding Burnout)

Do not leave the test too early. Carefully review your answers if possible.

Pacing and endurance are important. Practice helps develop both. Even though a number of examinees may leave an examination session early, especially in the last session of the last day, do not leave prematurely. Use any extra time at the end to return to unresolved questions or carefully recheck your answers. Do not be too casual in your review or you may overlook serious mistakes. Many students report that near the end of a booklet they suddenly remember facts that help answer questions they had guessed on earlier.

Remember your goals, and keep in mind the effort you have devoted to studying compared with the small additional effort needed to complete and check over the examination. Every point you earn is to your advantage. The difference between passing and an average score is far fewer questions than you might think. About 25% of students who failed were within 15 questions of passing.

Do not panic if you are unfamiliar with a particular photograph.

The "Glossy" Booklet

The "glossy" booklets contain many questions with accompanying gross and microscopic photographs. Two such booklets appeared in the June 1995 exam.

Student experience shows that many of these questions can be answered correctly independent of the photograph.

Types of photographs include gross pathology (e.g., hydatidiform mole, cardiac valve vegetations), histopathology (e.g., liver cirrhosis, myocardial infarction, glomerulonephritis), blood smears (e.g., target cells, basophilic stippling), dermatopathology (e.g., lupus, Lyme disease, basal cell carcinoma), and imaging (e.g., CT anatomy, cerebral angiogram, plain film fractures).

TESTING AGENCIES

National Board of Medical Examiners (NBME)
Department of Testing Services
3930 Chestnut Street
Philadelphia, PA 19104
(215) 590-9700

Educational Commission for Foreign Medical Graduates
3624 Market Street, Fourth Floor
Philadelphia, PA 19104-2685
(215) 386-5900 or (202) 293-9320
Fax: (215) 386-9196

Federation of State Medical Boards
400 Fuller Wiser Road, Suite 300
Euless, TX 76039-3855
(817) 868-4000
Fax: (817) 868-4099

REFERENCES

1. Bidese, Catherine M., *U.S. Medical Licensure Statistics and Current Licensure Requirements 1995,* American Medical Association, 1995 (ISBN 0899707270).
2. National Board of Medical Examiners, *Part I Examination Guidelines and Sample Items, 1991,* Philadelphia, 1990.
3. National Board of Medical Examiners, *Bulletin of Information and Description of National Board Examinations, 1991,* Philadelphia, 1990.
4. Federation of State Medical Boards and National Board of Medical Examiners, *United States Medical Licensing Examination: 1995 Step 1 General Instructions, Content Outline, and Sample Items,* Philadelphia, 1994.
5. Federation of State Medical Boards and National Board of Medical Examiners, *United States Medical Licensing Examination: 1995 Bulletin of Information,* Philadelphia, 1994.

6. "Report on 1994 Examinations," *The National Board Examiner,* Winter 1995, Vol. 42, No. 1, pp. 1–4.

7. National Board of Medical Examiners, *Performance Norms for the June 1994 USMLE Step 1,* Philadelphia, 1994.

8. "Highlights of the 1991 Annual Meeting: Standard Setting System, Score Reporting and Examinee Feedback Plan, USMLE Implementation Plans," *The National Board Examiner,* Spring 1991, Vol. 38, No. 2, pp. 1–6.

9. Swanson, David B., Case, Susan M., Melnick, Donald E., et al., "Impact of the USMLE Step 1 on Teaching and Learning of the Basic Biomedical Sciences," *Academic Medicine,* September Supplement 1992, Vol. 67, No. 9, pp. 553–556.

10. O'Donnell, M.J., Obenshain, S. Scott, and Erdmann, James B, "I: Background Essential to the Proper Use of Results of Step 1 and Step 2 of the USMLE," *Academic Medicine,* October 1993, Vol. 68, No. 10, pp. 734–739.

11. "Report on 1994 Examinations," *op. cit.,* Vol. 4, No. 1, pp. 1–4.

12. National Board of Medical Examiners, *Summary of Examinee Performance,* Philadelphia, 1995.

13. FSMB and NBME, *USMLE: 1993 Step 1 General Instructions, Content Outline, and Sample Items, op. cit.*

14. Swanson, *op. cit.*

15. Iserson, K., *Getting into Residency,* Tucson, AZ, Galen Press, 1993 (ISBN 1883620104).

16. Case, Susan M., and Swanson, David B., "Validity of NBME Part I and Part II Scores for Selection of Residents in Orthopaedic Surgery, Dermatology, and Preventive Medicine," *Academic Medicine,* February Supplement 1993, Vol. 68, No. 2, pp. S51–S56.

17. FSMB and NBME, *USMLE: 1993 Step 1 General Instructions, Content Outline, and Sample Items, op. cit.*

18. Swanson, *op. cit.*

19. "Report on 1994 Examinations," *op. cit.*

20. National Board of Medical Examiners, *United States Medical Licensing Examination: 1993 Application Instructions for Step 1 and Step 2,* Philadelphia, 1992.

21. "Report on 1994 Examinations," *op. cit.*

22. Swanson, *op. cit..*

23. Robinson, Adam, *What Smart Students Know,* New York, Crown Publishers, 1993 (ISBN 0517880857).

24. National Board Examinations, "Preliminary Report on June 1988 Part I Performance," *The National Board Examiner,* Fall 1988, Vol. 35, No. 4, p. 3.

25. O'Donnell, *op. cit.*

Special Situations

First Aid for the International Medical Graduate

First Aid for the Osteopathic Medical Student

International Medical Graduate (IMG) is the term now used to describe any student or graduate of a non-US or non-Canadian medical school, no matter whether he or she is a US citizen or not. The old term Foreign Medical Graduate (FMG) has been replaced because it was misleading when applied to US citizens attending medical schools outside the US.

The IMG's Steps to Licensure in the US

In order to become licensed to practice in the US, the IMG must go through the following steps (not necessarily in this order). These steps must be completed by all IMGs even if you are already a practicing physician and have completed a residency program in your own country:

- Complete the basic sciences program of your medical school (equivalent to the first two years of US medical school).
- Take the USMLE Step 1. You can do this while still in school or after graduating, but your medical school must certify that you have completed the basic science part of your school's curriculum in order to be eligible.
- Complete the clinical clerkship program of your medical school (equivalent to the third and fourth years of US medical school).
- Take the USMLE Step 2. If you are still in medical school, you must be certified by your school that you are within one year of graduating to be allowed to take Step 2.
- Take the Educational Commission for Foreign Medical Graduates (ECFMG) English test (or an equivalent to the Test of English as a Foreign Language recognized by the ECFMG).
- Graduate with your medical degree.
- Once you have passed Step 1, Step 2, and the English test, you must obtain an ECFMG certificate; you can get this from ECFMG (see below) after you have sent them a copy of your degree, which they will verify with your medical school. This can take eight weeks or more. The ECFMG certificate is required for you to obtain a position in an accredited residency program; some programs will not even allow you to apply unless you already have this certificate.
- Starting mid-1996 or early 1997 it will also be necessary to pass the Clinical Skills Assessment (CSA) exam (see below) in order to obtain an ECFMG certificate.
- Apply for residency positions in your field of interest, either directly or through the National Residency Matching Program ("the Match"). You do not need to have an ECFMG certificate, to have graduated, or to have passed any USMLE Step or the English test in order to apply for residencies, either directly or through the Match, but you do need to have passed

all the examinations necessary for ECFMG certification (i.e., Step 1, Step 2, English test) by a certain deadline (in 1996, this is February 23) in order to be entered into the Match itself. If you have not passed all these exams, you will be automatically withdrawn from the Match.

- Obtain a visa to allow you to enter and work in the US if you are not already a US citizen or green card holder (permanent resident).

- Some states require IMGs to obtain an educational/training/limited medical license that allows them to practice as a resident in the state where their residency program is located. The residency program may assist you with this application. Note that medical licensing is the prerogative of each individual state, not of the federal government, and that states vary in the exact laws about licensing (although all 50 US states recognize the USMLE).

- Take USMLE Step 3 during your residency, and then obtain a full medical license. Note that as an IMG you will not be able to take Step 3 and obtain an independent license until you have completed one or two years of residency, depending on which state you are in. However, even if you live in a state that requires two or three years of residency in order to take Step 3, you can still take Step 3 and then obtain a license in another state. Once you have a license in any one state you are permitted to practice in federal facilities such as VA hospitals and in Indian Health Service facilities in any state. This can open the door to "moonlighting" opportunities. For details on individual state rules, write to the licensing board in the state in question or contact FSMB (see below).

- Complete your residency, and then take the appropriate specialty board exams in order to become board certified (e.g., in internal medicine, surgery, etc.). If you already have a specialty certification in your home country (e.g., in surgery, cardiology), some specialty boards may grant you six months' or one year's credit toward your total residency time.

USMLE Step 1 and the IMG

The USMLE Step 1 is administered by the ECFMG at 78 examination centers in North America and around the world in June and September of each year. USMLE Step 1 is often the first, and for most IMGs the most challenging, hurdle to overcome. The USMLE is a standardized licensing system that gives IMGs a level playing field (it is the same exam series taken by US graduates, even though it is administered by the ECFMG rather than by the NBME). This means that pass marks for IMGs, for both Step 1 and Step 2, are determined by a statistical process that is based on the scores of US medical students in 1991. In general, to pass Step 1, you will probably have to score higher than the bottom 8–10% of US and Canadian graduates in Step 1. However, in 1994 only 51% of ECFMG candidates passed Step 1 on their first attempt, compared with 91% of US and Canadian graduates.

A good Step 1 score is key to a strong IMG application.

As an IMG, you must do as well as you can on Step 1 in particular. Probably nobody ever feels totally ready to take Step 1, but nearly all IMGs require a period of serious study and preparation to reach their potential. A poor score on Step 1 will be a distinct disadvantage when applying for most residencies. Remember that if you pass Step 1, you cannot retake it to try to improve your score. Your goals should be to beat the mean, since you can then confidently assert that you have done better than average for US students. Good Step 1 scores lend credibility to your residency application.

Do commercial review courses help improve your scores? Reports vary, and these courses can be expensive. Many IMGs decide to try USMLE on their own first and then consider a review course only if they fail. But many states require that you pass within three attempts, so you do not have many chances. (For more information on review courses, see pp. 259–263.)

The Other Exams and the IMG

- **USMLE Step 2.** In the past, this examination has had a reputation for being much easier than Step 1, but this no longer seems to be the case for both IMGs and US medical students. In 1994, 47% of ECFMG candidates passed on their first attempt, compared with 92% of US and Canadian candidates. Since this is a clinical sciences exam, cultural and geographical considerations play a greater role than they do in Step 1. For example, if your medical education gave you a lot of exposure to malaria, brucellosis and malnutrition but little to alcohol withdrawal, child abuse, and cholesterol screening, you will need to do some work to familiarize yourself with topics that are more heavily emphasized in US medicine. Also, you will need to have a basic understanding of the legal and social context of US medicine, because you will be asked questions about communicating with and advising patients.

Native English-speaking IMGs are also required to take the language test.

- **The English language test.** All IMGs must take an English test, irrespective of citizenship (including US-born US citizens) and native language. Though this exam can appear absurd to the native English speaker, it is generally considered to be a fair and appropriate test. It does not involve any use of medical knowledge or medical terminology; in the first part, candidates listen to tape recordings of typical English conversations and are asked simple questions to assess their comprehension. In the second part, written sentences are presented in which candidates are asked to choose an appropriate replacement for a missing word that is both grammatically correct and meaningful. This test is strictly pass-fail; there is no numerical grade. If English is not your native language, you must assess your English ability. The test is generally not difficult for those who feel comfortable having ordinary, natural conversations with Americans. Having lived in or visited the US for an extended period is almost always an advantage for the foreign-born IMG seeking US licensure.

There is a big difference between textbook learning of a language and actually being immersed in the culture that goes with it.

■ **Clinical Skills Assessment (CSA).** This is a new requirement that will be instituted starting mid- to late 1996. In the CSA, candidates will be required to demonstrate their skills in history taking, physical examination, English language communication, and interviewing in the course of ten half-hour interactions with each of ten standardized "patients" all of whom are specially trained actors. The exam will last five hours and will be conducted over an entire morning or an entire afternoon session. Each "patient" will grade each student. The interaction will not be watched by any observers, but it will be video- and audio-taped in case any problems or disputes arise later. In order to take the CSA, you must already have passed USMLE Steps 1 and 2 and the English language test. You will need to have passed the CSA to enter the residency Match.

According to current plans, the CSA will not be offered outside the United States, but it will be offered almost all year round at a continually rotating set of locations in the US, with between 20 and 40 candidates being examined at each site each day. Applicants will be offered a choice of sites and dates where they can take the exam, but clearly the more flexible you are about your choice of site, the easier it will be to schedule the exam without excessive waiting periods. Unfortunately, this will be an expensive exam. The ECFMG anticipates that the fee will be around $700–$750.

Passing this exam demonstrates your ability to use English in the practice of clinical medicine with patients. This exam will require that you demonstrate proficiency in English conversation in the context of doctor-patient encounters. Fluency, intelligible pronunciation, and organized history and physical exam skills are likely to be keys to success.

Resources for the IMG

■ ECFMG
3624 Market Street, Fourth Floor
Philadelphia, PA 19104-2685
(215) 386-5900 or (202) 293-9320
Fax: (215) 386-9196

This number is answered only between 9:00 am and 12:30 pm, and between 1:30 pm and 5:00 pm Monday through Friday EST. ECFMG often takes a long time to answer the phone and is often busy at peak times of the year, and there is then a long voice-mail message to listen to, so it is better to write or fax early rather than rely on a last-minute phone call. Don't contact the National Board of Medical Examiners. All IMG exam affairs are conducted by ECFMG. ECFMG publishes the *Handbook for Foreign Medical Graduates* and *Information Booklet* on ECFMG certification and the USMLE program; the latter gives details of dates and locations of forthcoming USMLE, CSA, and English tests for IMGs, together with application forms. It is free of charge and is also available from public affairs offices of US embassies and consulates worldwide, as well as from Overseas Educational Advisory Centers.

■ Federation of State Medical Boards

400 Fuller Wiser Road, Suite 300

Euless, TX 76039-3855

(817) 868-4000

Fax: (817) 868-4099

FSMB publishes Exchange, Section I, which gives detailed information on examination and licensing requirements in all US jurisdictions. The 1995–1996 edition costs $25 (1995 price; subject to change). Texas residents must add 7.75% state sales tax. To obtain publications, write to Federation Publications at the above address. All orders must be prepaid by cashier's check or money order payable to the Federation. Personal checks are not accepted. Foreign orders must be accompanied by an international money order or the equivalent, payable in US dollars through a US bank or a US affiliate of a foreign bank.

■ Some of the Step 1 commercial review courses listed in Section III are conducted outside the US. Write or call the course providers for details.

■ The Internet newsgroups misc.education.medical and bit.listserv.medforum can be valuable forums to exchange information about licensing exams, residency applications and so on.

FIRST AID FOR THE OSTEOPATHIC MEDICAL STUDENT

NBOME Part I—The Basics

The National Board of Osteopathic Medicine Examination (NBOME) is the osteopathic version of the USMLE. Osteopathic students must pass Parts I and II in order to graduate. In 1995, the NBOME introduced a new assessment tool called the Comprehensive Osteopathic Medical Licensing Examination (COMLEX). Like the NBOME that it will replace, COMLEX is to be administered in three Levels. The new examinations will be phased over a three-year period (Figure 12). In 1995, only the Level III exam was administered, by 1997 all three levels of COMLEX will be administered. COMLEX will then be the only exam offered. A stated goal of this program is to get all states to recognize this examination as equivalent to the USMLE and to allow DO candidates to use this examination for licensing.

Like the Step 1, the NBOME Part I is a multiple-choice examination given over two days. It consists of four booklets, each containing approximately 150 questions. You are allotted 240 minutes for each booklet. In order to sit for Level I, you must have successfully completed at least 75% of the second-year curriculum.

FIGURE 12. Test Dates for NBOME and COMLEX

1996	Part I	NBOME	June 4–5 October 15–16
	Level II	COMLEX	March 12–13 October 15–16
	Level III	COMLEX	February 18–19 June 11–12
1997	Level I	COMLEX	June 3–4 October 14–15
	Level II	COMLEX	March 11–12 October 14–15
	Level III	COMLEX	February 18–19 June 10–11

The exam consists of one-best-answer questions, negatively phrased best answer questions, and matching sets. Questions are often organized with clinical case vignettes that consist of short cases with three to six associated questions. In the June 1995 administration of the NBOME Part I, there were approximately seven clinical vignettes per booklet. In addition to the seven traditional basic science subjects covered by the USMLE Step 1, the NBOME Part I also tests osteopathic principles.

For all three Levels, raw scores are converted to a score ranging from 5 to 995. For Part I and Level II, a score of 400 is required to pass. For Level III, a score of 350 is required. The COMLEX will use the same conversion scales. Scores are usually mailed eight weeks after the test date. In 1995, 88% of all first-takers passed the June administration of the NBOME Part I. The mean score on the June 1995 exam was 488. If you pass an NBOME or COMLEX examination, you are not allowed to retake that test to improve your grade. If you fail, there is no limit to the number of times you can retake the exam in an effort to pass.

NBOME and the USMLE

Aside from dealing with the NBOME Part I, you must decide if you will also take the USMLE Step 1. We recommend that you consider taking the USMLE in addition to the NBOME for the following reasons:

■ **If you are applying to allopathic residencies.** Though there is growing acceptance of NBOME certification by allopathic residencies, some allopathic programs prefer or require passage of the USMLE Step 1. These include academic programs and programs in competitive specialties. Fourth-year DO students who have already matched can tell you what programs and specialties are looking for USMLE scores.

- **If you plan to practice in Texas, Louisiana, or North Carolina.** These states require that osteopathic physicians pass the USMLE system to obtain a license for practice. However, these states may also have reciprocating agreements with other states that accept the NBOME. There, you might be licensed in another state and then petition to have your license transferred.
- **If you are unsure regarding your postgraduate training plans.** Certainly, successful passage of both the NBOME Part I and USMLE Step 1 will provide you with the greatest range of options when applying for internship and residency training.

Unfortunately, taking both exams can be a trying ordeal. Students planning to take both exams in June 1996 have to deal with the USMLE Step 1 one week after taking the NBOME Part I. In October Step 1 and Part I examination dates conflict. An alternative would be to take Part I or Step 1 in June and wait till October to sit for the other exam. The clinical classwork that most DO students receive during the summer of their third year (as opposed to starting clinical clerkships) is considered helpful in integrating the basic science knowledge for the NBOME or the USMLE.

Preparing for the NBOME

Student experience suggests that you should start studying for the NBOME four to six months before the test date. An early start would allow you to devote up to a month per subject. The recommendations made in Section I regarding study and testing methods, strategies and resources hold true for the NBOME as well. In addition, you should seek resources to review osteopathic principles such as the Student Osteopathic Medical Association's "blue book" or Greenman's *Principles of Manual Medicine*. The SOMA blue book has been out of print for several years, so get a copy from a third-year student. Take full advantage of the *Examination Guidelines and Sample Exam* distributed by the NBOME. This publication and additional information can be obtained by writing:

NBOME
2700 River Road, Suite 607
Des Plaines, IL 60018

Apart from the osteopathic principles, the NBOME and the USMLE exams are similar in scope, content, and emphasis. Both exams often require that you to apply and integrate knowledge over several areas of basic science in order to answer a question. Likewise, your preparation for both exams will be very similar. However, students who have taken both exams report that the NBOME makes greater use of "buzzwords" (e.g., rose spots in typhoid fever), whereas the USMLE often avoids buzzwords in favor of straight descriptions of clinical findings or symptoms (e.g., rose-colored papules on the abdomen instead of rose spots).

Database of High-Yield Facts

Anatomy
Behavioral Science
Biochemistry
Microbiology
Pathology
Pharmacology
Physiology

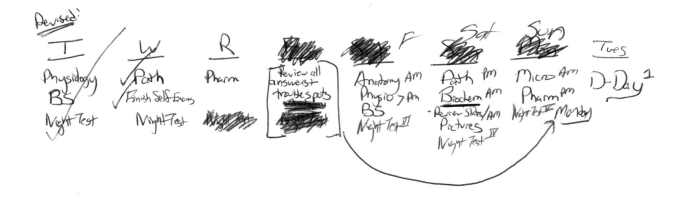

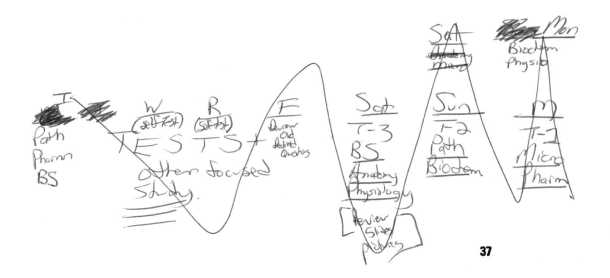

The 1996 edition of *First Aid for the USMLE Step 1* contains a revised and expanded database of basic science material that student authors and faculty have identified as high-yield for boards review. The facts are loosely organized according to the seven traditional basic medical science disciplines (anatomy, behavioral science, biochemistry, microbiology, pathology, pharmacology, and physiology). Each discipline is then divided into smaller subsections of related facts. Individual facts are generally presented in a three-column format, with the **Title** of the fact in the first column, the **Description** of the fact in the second column, and the **Mnemonic** or **Special Note** in the third column.

Some facts do not have a mnemonic and are presented in a two-column format. Others are presented in list or tabular form in order to emphasize key associations. The database structure is useful for reviewing material already learned. This section is not ideal for learning complex or highly conceptual material for the first time. At the end of each basic science section we list supplementary high-yield topics to help focus your additional review.

The Database of High-Yield Facts is not comprehensive. Use it to complement your core study material and not as your primary study source. The facts and notes have been condensed and edited to emphasize the essential material, and as a result each entry is "incomplete." Work with the material, add your own notes and mnemonics, and realize that not all memory techniques work for all students.

We update Section II annually to keep current with new trends in boards content as well as to expand our base of high-yield information. However, we must note that inevitably many other very-high-yield entries and topics are not yet included in our database.

We actively encourage medical students and faculty to submit entries and mnemonics so that we may enhance the database for future students. We also solicit recommendations of alternate tools for study that may be useful in preparing for the examination, such as diagrams, charts, and computer-based tutorials. (*See* How to Contribute, page xiii.)

Disclaimer

These entries reflect student opinions of what is high-yield. Owing to the diverse sources of material, no attempt has been made to individually trace or reference the origins of entries. We have regarded mnemonics as essentially in the public domain. All errors and omissions will be gladly corrected if brought to the attention of the authors, either through the publisher or directly by e-mail.

Anatomy

A large number of topics fall under this heading, which includes gross anatomy, embryology, neuroanatomy, and histology. Studying all anatomy topics in great detail is generally a low-yield approach. However, do not ignore anatomy altogether. Review what you have already learned and what you wish you had learned. Don't memorize all the small details. Some questions will require you to identify a structure on anatomical cross section, electron micrograph, or photomicrograph.

When studying, try to stress clinically important material. For example, be familiar with gross anatomy that is related to traumatic injuries (e.g., fractures), procedures (e.g., lumbar puncture), and common surgeries (e.g., cholecystectomy). There are also several questions on the exam involving x-rays, CT scans, and MR scans. Focus on learning the basic anatomy at key levels in the body (e.g., sagittal brain MRI, axial CT midthorax, abdomen and pelvis). Basic neuroanatomy, especially pathways, has good yield. Basic embryology has moderate yield and is worth reviewing.

Cell Type
Embryology
Gross Anatomy
Histology
Neuroanatomy
High-Yield Topics

Erythrocyte

Anucleate, biconcave → large surface area: volume ratio → easy gas exchange (O_2 and CO_2). Source of energy = glucose (90% anaerobically degraded to lactate, 10% by HMP shunt). Survival time = 120 days. Membrane contains the chloride-bicarbonate antiport important in the "physiologic chloride shift," which allows the RBC to transport CO_2 from the periphery to the lungs for elimination.

Eryth = red
Erythrocytosis = Polycythemia
= increased number of red cells
Anisocytosis = varying sizes
Poikilocytosis = varying shapes
Reticulocyte = baby erythrocyte

Leukocyte

Types: granulocytes (basophils, eosinophils, neutrophils) and mononuclear cells (lymphocytes, monocytes). Responsible for defense against infections. Normally 4,000–10,000 per microliter.

Leuk = white.

Basophil

Mediates allergic reaction. <1% of all leukocytes. Bilobate nucleus. Densely basophilic granules containing heparin (anticoagulant), histamine (vasodilator) and other vasoactive amines, and SRS-A (**S**low-**R**eacting **S**ubstance of **A**naphylaxis).

Mast cell

Mediates allergic reaction. Degranulation = release of histamine, heparin, and eosinophil chemotactic factors. Can bind IgE to membrane. Mast cells resemble basophils structurally and functionally but are not the same cell type.

Masten = fatten.
Involved in Type I hypersensitivity reactions. Cromolyn sodium prevents mast cell degranulation.

Eosinophil

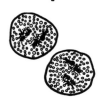

1%–6% of all leukocytes. Bilobate nucleus. Packed with large eosinophilic granules of uniform size. Defends against helminthic and protozoan infections. Highly phagocytic for antigen-antibody complexes.

Eosinophilic = eosin loving.
N = neoplastic
A = asthma
A = allergic processes
C = collagen vascular diseases
P = parasites

Neutrophil

Acute inflammatory response cell. 40%–75% WBCs. Phagocytic. Multilobed nucleus. Large, spherical, azurophilic 1° granules (called lysosomes) contain hydrolytic enzymes, lysozyme, myeloperoxidase.

Hypersegmented polys are seen in vit. B_{12}/folate deficiency.

Monocyte	2%–10% of leukocytes. Large. Kidney-shaped nucleus. Extensive "frosted glass" cytoplasm. Differentiates into macrophages in tissues.	
Lymphocyte	Small. Round, densely staining nucleus. Small amount of pale cytoplasm. B lymphocytes produce antibodies. T lymphocytes manifest the cellular immune response as well as regulate B lymphocytes and macrophages.	
B lymphocyte	Part of humoral immune response. Arises from stem cells in bone marrow. Matures in marrow. Migrates to peripheral lymphoid tissue (follicles of lymph nodes, white pulp of spleen, unencapsulated lymphoid tissue). When antigen is encountered, B cells produce Ab. Has memory. Can function as antigen-presenting cell (APC).	**B** = **B**one marrow or **B**ursa of Fabricius (in birds).
T lymphocyte	Mediates cellular immune response. Originates from stem cells in the bone marrow, but matures in the thymus. T cells differentiate into cytotoxic T cells (MHC I, CD8), helper T cells (MHC II, CD4), suppressor T cells, delayed hypersensitivity T cells.	**T** is for **T**hymus. **CD** is for **C**luster of **D**ifferentiation. $MHC \times CD = 8$ (e.g., $2 \times 4 = 8$).
Macrophage	Phagocytizes bacteria, cell debris, and senescent red cells and scavenges damaged cells and tissues. Long life in tissues. Macrophages differentiate from circulating blood monocytes. Activated by γ-IFN. Can function as APC.	*Macrophage* = large eater.
Airway cells	Ciliated cells extend to the respiratory bronchioles; mucous cells extend only to the terminal bronchioles. Type I cells (97% of alveolar surfaces) line the alveoli. Type II cells (3%) secrete pulmonary surfactant (dipalmitoylphosphatidylcholine), which lowers the alveolar surface tension.	All the mucus secreted can be swept orally (ciliated cells run deeper). A lecithin:sphingomyelin ratio of > 1.5 in amniotic fluid is indicative of fetal lung maturity.

Juxtaglomerular apparatus (JGA)

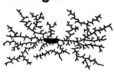

JGA = JG cells (modified smooth muscle of afferent arteriole) and macula densa (Na⁺ sensor, part of the distal convoluted tubule). JG cells secrete renin (leading to ↑ angiotensin II and aldosterone levels) in response to ↓ renal blood pressure, ↓ Na⁺ delivery to distal tubule, and ↑ sympathetic tone. JG cells also secrete erythropoietin.

JGA defends glomerular filtration rate via the renin-angiotensin system.
Juxta = close by.

Microglia

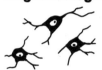

CNS phagocytes. Mesodermal origin. Not readily discernible in Nissl stains. Have small irregular nuclei and relatively little cytoplasm. In response to tissue damage, transform into large amoeboid phagocytic cells.

HIV-infected microglia fuse to form multinucleated giant cells in the CNS.

Oligodendroglia

Function to myelinate multiple CNS axons. In Nissl stains, they appear as small nuclei with dark chromatin and little cytoplasm. Predominant type of glial cell in white matter.

These are the cells that are destroyed in multiple sclerosis.

Schwann cells

Function to myelinate PNS axons. Unlike oligodendroglia, many Schwann cells myelinate a single PNS axon.

Schwannomas are commonly seen in neurofibromatosis.

Cones

For bright, acute vision (color, concentrated in fovea). Comprise inner and outer segments connected by 9 + 0 modified cilium; outer segment disks continuous with plasma membrane. Contain iodopsin pigment, red-green-blue specific.

Cones are for Color, and their outer segments are Continuous (with the plasma membrane, unlike rods).
Cones have a sharp tip (acuity).

Rods

For night vision (no color; many more than cones; none in the fovea). Comprise inner and outer segments connected by 9 + 0 modified cilium; outer segment disks not continuous with plasma membrane. Rods contain rhodopsin pigment.

Rods have Rhodopsin.
Rods have a high sensitivity due to multiple rods synapsing on one bipolar cell (convergence).

ANATOMY—EMBRYOLOGY

Umbilical cord

Contains 2 umbilical arteries, which return deoxygenated blood from the fetus, and 1 umbilical vein that supplies oxygenated blood from the placenta to the fetus.

Embryologic derivatives

Ectoderm	Epidermis (including hair, nails), nervous system, adrenal medulla.
Mesoderm	Connective tissue, muscle, bone, cardiovascular structures, lymphatics, urogenital structures, and serous linings of body cavities (e.g., peritoneal), spleen.
Endoderm	Gut tube epithelium and derivatives (e.g., lungs, liver, pancreas).
Notochord	Nucleus pulposus of the intervertebral disc.

Rule of 2's for 2nd week of development

2 germ layers (bilaminar disc): epiblast/hypoblast

2 cavities (amniotic, yolk sac)

2 components to "placenta" (cytotrophoblast, syncytiotrophoblast)

Neural crest derivatives

ANS, dorsal root ganglia, melanocytes, chromaffin cell of adrenal medulla, enterochromaffin cells, pia, celiac ganglion, Schwann cells, odontoblasts, parafollicular cells (of thyroid).

Dura is of mesodermal origin.

Aortic arch derivatives

1st = part of maxillary artery.

2nd = stapedial artery and hyoid artery.

3rd = common carotid artery and proximal part of internal carotid artery.

4th = on left, aortic arch; on right, proximal part of right subclavian artery.

6th = proximal part of pulmonary arteries and (on left only) ductus arteriosus.

4th arch (4 limbs) = systemic.
6th arch = pulmonary and the pulmonary to systemic shunt (ductus arteriosus).

Fetal erythropoiesis

Fetal erythropoiesis occurs in
1. Yolk sac (3–8 wk)
2. Liver (6–30 wk)
3. Spleen (9 wk–28 wks)
4. Bone marrow (28 wks onward)

Fetal-postnatal derivatives

1. Umbilical vein—ligamentum teres hepatis
2. Umbilical arteries—medial umbilical ligaments
3. Ductus arteriosus—ligamentum arteriosum
4. Ductus venosus—ligamentum venosum
5. Foramen ovale—fossa ovalis
6. Allantois—urachus—median umbilical ligament

Branchial apparatus

Branchial clefts are derived from ectoderm.
Branchial arches are derived from mesoderm and neural crests.
Branchial pouches are derived from endoderm.

CAP covers outside from inside (Clefts = ectoderm, Arches = mesoderm, Pouches = endoderm)

Branchial arch 1 derivatives	Meckel's cartilage: mandible, malleus, incus, sphenomandibular ligament. Muscles: muscles of mastication (temporalis, masseter, lateral and medial pterygoids), mylohyoid, anterior belly of digastric, tensor tympani, tensor veli palatini. Nerve: CN V_3	
Branchial arch 2 derivatives	Reichert's cartilage: stapes, styloid process, lesser horn of hyoid, stylohyoid ligament. Muscles: muscles of facial expression—stapedius, stylohyoid, posterior belly of digastric. Nerve: CN VII	
Branchial arch 3 derivatives	Cartilage: greater horn of hyoid. Muscles: stylopharyngeus. Nerve: CN IX	Think of pharynx: stylo**pharyngeus** innervated by glosso**pharyngeal** nerve.
Branchial arches 4 to 6 derivatives	Cartilages: thyroid, cricoid, arytenoids, corniculate, cuneiform. Muscles (4th arch): most pharyngeal constrictors, cricothyroid, levator veli palatini. Muscles (6th arch): intrinsic muscles of larynx. Nerve: 4th arch–X 6th arch–X (recurrent laryngeal branch)	Arch 5 makes no major developmental contributions.
Branchial arch innervation	Arch 1 derivatives supplied by CN V_2 and V_3. Arch 2 derivatives supplied by CN VII. Arch 3 derivatives supplied by CN IX. Arch 4 derivatives supplied by CN X.	
Branchial cleft derivatives	1st cleft develops into external auditory meatus. 2nd through 4th clefts form temporary cervical sinuses, which are obliterated by proliferation of 2nd arch mesenchyme.	Persistent cervical sinus can lead to a branchial cyst in the neck.

Ear development		
Bones	**Muscles**	**Miscellaneous**
Incus/malleus–1st arch Stapes–2nd arch	Tensor tympani (V_3)–1st arch Stapedius (VII)–2nd arch	External auditory meatus–1st cleft Eardrum, eustachian tube–1st pouch

44

Pharyngeal pouch derivatives	1st pouch develops into middle ear cavity, eustachian tube, mastoid air cells. 2nd pouch develops into epithelial lining of palatine tonsil. 3rd pouch (dorsal wings) develops into inferior parathyroids. 3rd pouch (ventral wings) develops into thymus. 4th pouch develops into superior parathyroids. 5th pouch develops into the ultimobranchial bodies, which become the C cells of the thyroid.	1st pouch contributes to endoderm-lined structures of ear. 3rd pouch contributes to 3 structures (thymus, L and R inferior parathyroids).
Thymus	Site of T-cell maturation. Encapsulated. From epithelium of 3rd branchial pouches. Lymphocytes of mesenchymal origin. Cortex is dense with immature T cells; medulla is pale with mature T cells and epithelial reticular cells. Positive and negative selection occurs at the cortico-medullary junction.	Think of the Thymus as "finishing school" for T cells. They arrive immature and "dense" in the cortex; they are mature in the medulla.
Thyroid development	Thyroid diverticulum arises from floor of primitive pharynx, descends into neck. Connected to tongue by thyroglossal duct, which normally disappears but may persist as pyramidal lobe of thyroid. Foramen cecum is normal remnant of thyroglossal duct.	
Tongue development	1st branchial arch forms anterior ⅔ (thus pain via CN V₃, taste via CN VII). 3rd and 4th arches form posterior ⅓ (thus pain and taste mainly via CN IX, extreme posterior via CN X). Motor innervation is via CN XII.	Taste is CN VII, IX, X. Motor is CN XII. Pain is CN V₃.
Cleft lip and cleft palate	Cleft lip—failure of fusion of the maxillary and medial nasal processes. Cleft palate—failure of fusion of the lateral palatine processes with each other, the nasal septum, and/or the median palatine process.	
Diaphragm embryology	Diaphragm is derived from: 1. Septum transversum 2. Pleuroperitoneal folds 3. Dorsal mesentery of esophagus 4. Body wall	

Heart embryology	**Embryonic structure**	**Gives rise to**
	Bulbus cordis	Right ventricle and aortic outflow tract
	Primitive ventricle	Left ventricle, except for the aortic outflow tract
	Truncus arteriosus	Ascending aorta and pulmonary trunk
	Primitive atria	Auricular appendages
	Left horn of sinus venosus	Coronary sinus
	Right horn of sinus venosus	Smooth part of the right atrium

Cyst/sinus/fistula/atresia

Cyst is a spherical epithelium-lined cavity.

Pseudocyst is a spherical cavity without epithelial lining.

Sinus is a blind-ending duct or space opening externally or internally.

Fistula is a patent (abnormal) canal with openings at both ends.

Atresia is a closure of a normal body opening or tubular organ.

Meckel's diverticulum

Persistence of the vitelline duct or yolk stalk. May contain ectopic acid-secreting gastric mucosa and/or pancreatic tissue. Most common congenital anomaly of the GI tract. Can cause bleeding or obstruction at the terminal ileum.

The five **2**'s:
2 inches long.
2 feet from the ileocecal valve.
2% of population.
Commonly presents in first **2** years of life.
May have **2** types of epithelia.

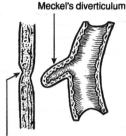

Meckel's diverticulum

Umbilicus

Pancreas embryology

Pancreas is derived from the foregut. Ventral pancreatic bud becomes pancreatic head, uncinate process (lower half of head), and main pancreatic duct. Dorsal pancreatic bud becomes body, tail, isthmus, and accessory pancreatic duct.

Associate "**vent**-ral" with main duct (a **vent** is a type of duct). Everything else comes from dorsal bud. Annular pancreas, a rare malformation, can cause duodenal obstruction.

Genital ducts

Mesonephric (wolffian) duct — Develops into epididymis, ductus deferens, ejaculatory duct, and seminal vesicles.

Paramesonephric (müllerian) duct — Develops into fallopian tube, uterus, and part of vagina.

Müllerian inhibiting substance secreted by testes suppresses development of male paramesonephric ducts.

Male/female genital homologues

Corpus spongiosum ≈ vestibular bulbs.
Bulbourethral glands (of Cowper) ≈ greater vestibular glands (of Bartholin).
Prostate gland ≈ urethral and paraurethral glands (of Skene).
Glans penis ≈ glans clitoris.
Ventral shaft of the penis ≈ labia minora.
Scrotum ≈ labia majora.

Congenital penile abnormalities

Hypospadias — Abnormal opening of penile urethra on inferior (ventral) side of penis due to failure of urethral folds to close.

Epispadias — Abnormal opening of penile urethra on superior (dorsal) side of penis due to faulty positioning of genital tubercle.

Exstrophy of the bladder is associated with epispadias.

Anatomy

HIGH-YIELD FACTS

Sperm development	Spermatogenesis: spermatogonia → 1° spermatocyte → 2° spermatocyte → spermatid → (spermiogenesis) → spermatozoa. Full development takes 2 months. Spermatogenesis in seminiferous tubules.
Derivation of sperm parts	Acrosome is derived from the Golgi apparatus, and flagellum (tail) from one of the centrioles. Middle piece (neck) has mitochondria.
Meiosis and ovulation	1° oocytes begin meiosis I during fetal life and complete meiosis I just prior to ovulation. Meiosis I is arrested in prophase for years until ovulation. Meiosis II is arrested in metaphase until fertilization.

Amniotic fluid abnormalities

Polyhydramnios	> 1.5–2 L of amniotic fluid; associated with esophageal/duodenal atresia, anencephaly
Oligohydramnios	< 0.5 L of amniotic fluid; associated with bilateral renal agenesis or posterior urethral valves (in males).

Potter's syndrome	Bilateral renal agenesis → oligohydramnios → limb deformities, facial deformities, pulmonary hypoplasia.

ANATOMY—GROSS ANATOMY

Erb-Duchenne palsy	Traction or tear of the superior trunk of the brachial plexus (C5 and C6 roots); follows fall to shoulder or trauma during delivery. Findings: Limb hangs by side, medially rotated (paralysis of lateral rotators), forearm is pronated (loss of biceps).	"Waiters's tip" owing to appearance of arm.
Lumbar puncture	CSF obtained from lumbar subarachnoid space between L4 and L5 (at the level of iliac crests). Structures pierced as follows: 1. Skin/superficial fascia 2. Ligaments (supraspinous, interspinous, ligamentum flavum) 3. Epidural space 4. Dura mater 5. Subdural space 6. Arachnoid 7. Subarachnoid space—CSF	
Radial nerve	Innervates posterior compartment of arm; extends elbow, supinates forearm, extends wrist and digits. Wraps around posterior of humerus in spiral groove with the deep brachial artery (vulnerable in fractures).	To *sup*inate is to move forearms as if carrying a bowl of *soup*. Lesion of radial nerve leads to wrist drop, "Saturday night palsy." Radial nerve is the great extender.

Nerve injury	Deficit in motion	Deficit in sensation
Radial	Triceps brachii (triceps reflex), anconeus, brachioradialis (brachioradialis reflex), and extensor carpi radialis longus	Posterior brachial cutaneous Dorsal antebrachial cutaneous
Median	No loss of power in any of the arm muscles; loss of forearm pronation, wrist flexion, finger flexion, and several thumb movements; eventually, thenar atrophy	Loss of sensation over the lateral palm and over the thumb and the radial 2½ fingers.
Ulnar	Impaired wrist flexion and adduction, and impaired adduction of thumb and the ulnar 2 fingers	
Axillary	Loss of deltoid action	
Musculocutaneous	Loss of function of coracobrachialis, biceps, and brachialis muscles (biceps reflex)	
Common peroneal	Loss of dorsiflexion (→ foot drop) +eversion • Common = foot drop	
Tibial	Loss of plantar flexion • Tibial → foot to Tibia	
Femoral	Loss of knee jerk • Femoral → knee jerk to groin	
Obturator	Loss of hip adduction • Obturator → hip adduction "obstruct c set"	

Recurrent laryngeal nerve	Supplies all intrinsic muscles of the larynx except the cricothyroid muscle. Left recurrent laryngeal nerve wraps around the arch of the aorta and the ligamentum arteriosum. Right recurrent laryngeal nerve wraps around right subclavian artery.	
Scalp and meninges: layers	Skin, Connective tissue, Aponeurosis, Loose connective tissue, Pericranium; skull; Dura mater, subdural space, Arachnoid, subarachnoid space, Pia mater, brain.	SCALP–skull–DsAsP. Also, mater = mother (protector) of the brain, pia = tender, dura = strong (durable). Loose connective tissue is vascular.
Spinal cord lower extent	In adults, spinal cord extends to lower border of L1-L2; subarachnoid space extends to lower border of S2. Lumbar puncture is usually performed in L3-L4 or L4-L5 interspaces, at level of cauda equina.	To keep the cord alive, keep the spinal needle between L3 and L5.
Spinal nerves	There are 31 spinal nerves altogether: 8 cervical, 12 thoracic, 5 lumbar, 5 sacral, 1 coccygeal.	31, just like 31 flavors!
Trigeminal ganglion	Also called semilunar ganglion or gasserian ganglion • Located in the trigeminal cave (of Meckel). Trigeminal neuralgia = tic douloureux	Trigeminal neuralgia can be treated with carbamazepine.

Landmark dermatomes	C2 is a posterior half of a skull "cap." C3 is a high turtleneck shirt. C4 is a low collar shirt. T4 is at the nipple. T7 is at the xyphoid process. T10 is at the umbilicus (important for early appendicitis pain referral). L1 is at the inguinal ligament. S2, S3, S4 erection and sensation of penile and anal zones.	L1 is IL (inguinal ligament). "S2, 3, 4 keeps the penis off the floor." Pain from the gallbladder may be referred to the right shoulder via the phrenic nerve.
Eight layers of abdominal wall/ spermatic cord	1. Skin 2. Fascia (Camper's and Scarpa's) → dartos muscle and fascia 3. External oblique → external spermatic fascia and superficial inguinal ring 4. Internal oblique → cremaster muscle and conjoint tendon 5. Transversus abdominis → no contribution except to conjoint tendon 6. Transversalis fascia → internal spermatic fascia and deep inguinal ring 7. Extraperitoneal fat 8. Peritoneum → tunica vaginalis testis and processus vaginalis	Scarpa's fascia is continuous with Colles' fascia of perineum.
Inguinal hernias Direct hernia Indirect hernia	Protrudes through the inguinal (Hesselbach's) triangle (bounded by inguinal ligament, inferior epigastric artery, and lateral border of rectus abdominis). Direct hernia bulges directly through abdominal wall medial to inferior epigastric artery. Goes through the superficial inguinal ring only. Indirect hernia goes through deep inguinal ring, superficial inguinal ring, and into scrotum. Due to failure of closure of processus vaginalis. Indirect hernia enters deep inguinal ring lateral to inferior epigastric artery.	
Mastication muscles	Three muscles close jaw: masseter, temporalis, medial pterygoid. One opens: lateral pterygoid. All are innervated by the trigeminal nerve (V_3).	Lateral Lowers (when speaking of pterygoids with respect to jaw motion).
Muscles with glossus	All muscles with root *glossus* in their names (except palatoglossus, innervated by vagus nerve) are innervated by hypo*glossal* nerve.	Palat—vagus nerve. *Glossus*—hypo*glossal* nerve.
Muscles with palat	All muscles with root *palat* in their names (except tensor veli palatini, innervated by mandibular branch of CN V) are innervated by vagus nerve.	Palat—vagus nerve (except tensor who was too tense).

Anatomy

HIGH-YIELD FACTS

Rotator cuff muscles	Shoulder muscles that form the rotator cuff: **S**upraspinatus, **I**nfraspinatus, teres minor, **S**ubscapularis.	**S I t S** (small t is for teres minor).
Thenar-hypothenar muscles	Thenar: **O**pponens pollicis, **A**bductor pollicis brevis, **F**lexor pollicis brevis. Hypothenar: **O**pponens digiti minimi, **A**bductor digiti minimi, **F**lexor digiti minimi.	Both groups perform the same functions: **O**ppose, **A**bduct, and **F**lex (**OAF**).
Unhappy triad/knee injury	This common football injury (caused by clipping from the side) consists of damage to medial collateral ligament, medial meniscus, and anterior cruciate ligament. Positive anterior drawer sign indicates tearing of the anterior cruciate ligament.	
Ligaments of the uterus	Pubocervical ligament, transverse cervical (cardinal) ligament, sacrocervical ligament, round ligament of uterus, round ligament of ovary. Round ligament of uterus is homologous (but not analogous) to gubernaculum testis: runs from labia majera to uterus. Round ligament of ovary runs from uterus to ovary.	
Carotid sheath	Three structures inside: 1. Internal jugular vein (lateral) 2. Common carotid artery (medial) 3. Vagus nerve (posterior)	**VAN**
Femoral sheath	Femoral sheath contains femoral artery, femoral vein, and femoral canal (containing deep inguinal lymph nodes). Femoral nerve lies outside femoral sheath.	Lateral to medial: **N-(AVEL)** = **N**erve–(**A**rtery–**V**ein–**E**mpty space–**L**ymphatics).
Broad ligament	Contains the round ligaments of the uterus, the uterine tubes, the ovarian ligaments, the epoophoron, and multiple lymphatic vessels and nerve fibers.	R U O E N *No Rule*
Diaphragm structures	Structures perforating diaphragm: At **T8**: IVC At **T10**: esophagus, vagus (two trunks) At **T12**: aorta (red), thoracic duct (white), azygous vein (blue) Diaphragm is innervated by **C3, 4,** and **5**. Pain from the diaphragm can be referred to the shoulder.	1-2-3 (number of items): 8 (IVC), 10 (esophagus, vagus), 12 (red-white-blue). **C3, 4, 5** keeps the diaphragm alive.
Portal-systemic anastomoses	Left gastric-azygous → *esophageal* varices. Superior-middle/inferior rectal → *hemorrhoids*. Paraumbilical-inferior epigastric → *caput* medusae (navel).	*Gut, butt*, and *caput*, the anastomoses 3. Commonly seen in alcoholic cirrhosis.
Bronchopulmonary segments	Each bronchopulmonary segment has a 3° (segmental) bronchus and two arteries (bronchial and pulmonary) in the center; veins and lymphatics drain along the borders.	Arteries run with Airways.

Lung relations	Right lung has three lobes, left has two lobes and lingula (homologue of right middle lobe). Right lung more common site for inhaled foreign body owing to less acute angle of right main stem bronchus.	Left lung is missing a lobe owing to space occupied by heart. The relation of the pulmonary artery to the bronchus at each lung hilus is described by **RALS**—Right Anterior; Left Superior
Pectinate line		
Above pectinate line	Internal hemorrhoids (not painful), adenocarcinoma, visceral innervation, blood supply, and lymphatic drainage.	Internal hemorrhoids receive visceral innervation. External hemorrhoids receive somatic innervation and are therefore painful.
Below pectinate line	External hemorrhoids (painful), squamous cell carcinoma, somatic innervation, blood supply, and lymphatic drainage.	
Autonomic innervation of the male sexual response	Erection is mediated by the parasympathetic nervous system. Emission is mediated by the sympathetic nervous system. Ejaculation is mediated by visceral and somatic nerves.	"Point and Shoot."
Ureters: course	Ureters pass **under** uterine artery and **under** ductus deferens (retroperitoneal).	Water (ureters) **under** the bridge (artery).
Clinically important landmarks	Pudendal nerve block—ischial spine. Appendix—⅔ of the way between umbilicus and anterior superior iliac spine (McBurney's point). Lumbar puncture—iliac crest.	

ANATOMY—HISTOLOGY

Special stains

Eosin	Acidic, anionic dye, binds acidophilic tissue with positive charge. Stains smooth ER.
Hematoxylin, methylene blue, toluidine blue	Basic, cationic dyes, bind basophilic nucleic acids with negative charge. Stains DNA, RNA, ribosomes, heparin-containing granules.
PAS	Stains glycogen and basement membranes.
Silver	Stains neuronal processes (Alzheimer's plaques, tangles) and reticular fibers. Also *Pneumocystis carinii* sporozoites and Legionellae.
Congo red	Amyloid (apple green birefringence under polarized light).
Prussian blue	Iron (think of Russia and the Iron Curtain).

Peripheral nerve layers

Endoneurium invests single nerve fiber.
Perineurium (permeability barrier) surrounds a fascicle of nerve fibers.
Epineurium (dense connective tissue) surrounds entire nerve (fascicles and blood vessels).

Perineurium = Permeability barrier, must be rejoined in microsurgery for limb reattachment.
Endo = inner.
Peri = around.
Epi = outer.

Meissner's corpuscles

Small, encapsulated sensory receptors found in dermis of palm, soles, and digits of skin. Involved in light discriminatory touch of glabrous (hairless) skin.

Pacinian corpuscles

Large, encapsulated sensory receptors found in deeper layers of skin at ligaments, joint capsules, serous membranes, mesenteries. Involved in pressure, coarse touch, vibration, and tension.

Choroid

Pigmented layer between the retina and sclera.
Functions:
1. Contains blood vessels that supply the retina.
2. Contains a dark pigment that absorbs stray light that passes beyond the retina.

Perilymph and endolymph

Perilymph (Na⁺ rich), similar to ECF, is in the osseous labyrinth; endolymph (K⁺ rich), similar to ICF, is in the membranous labyrinth.

Peri—think outside of cell (Na⁺).
Endo—think inside of cell (K⁺).
Endolymph is made by the stria vascularis.

Enteric plexuses

Myenteric

Also known as Auerbach's plexus. Contains cell bodies of some parasympathetic terminal effector neurons. Located between inner and outer layers of smooth muscle in GI tract wall.

Think of Auerbach, the quarterback (Staubach), a (muscular) football player.

Submucosal

Also known as Meissner's plexus. Contains cell bodies of some parasympathetic terminal effector neurons. Located between mucosa and inner layer of smooth muscle in GI tract wall.

Collagen types

Type I: bone, tendon, skin, dentin, fascia, late wound repair.
Type II: cartilage (including hyaline), vitreous body, nucleus pulposus.
Type III (reticulin): skin, blood vessels, uterus, fetal tissue, granulation tissue.
Type IV: basement membrane or basal lamina.

Anatomy

HIGH-YIELD FACTS

Epidermis layers	From base to surface: stratum Germinativum, stratum Spinosum, stratum Granulosum, stratum Lucidum, stratum Corneum.	**Good Students Give Loving Care.**
Bone matrix	Inorganic salts in bone are formed from calcium phosphate reordered as hydroxyapatite.	
Glomerular basement membrane	Formed from fused endothelial and podocyte basement membranes and coated with negatively charged heparan sulfate. Responsible for actual filtration of plasma according to net charge and size.	In **nephrotic syndrome negative charge is lost** (and plasma protein is lost in urine as a consequence).
Cilia structure	9 + 2 arrangement of microtubules. Peripheral 9 are unconventional. Central 2 are conventional. Dynein is an ATPase that links peripheral 9 doublets and causes bending of cilium by differential sliding of doublets.	9 + 2 arrangement. Kartagener's syndrome is due to a dynein arm defect, resulting in immotile cilia.
Intermediate filament	Permanent structure. Long fibrous molecules with 10-nm diameter. Linked to plasma membrane at desmosomes by desmoplakin. Very insoluble. No cytoplasmic pool of monomeric subunits. Intermediate filaments are tissue specific.	

Epithelial cells	Contain cytokeratin.
Connective tissue	Contains vimentin.
Muscle cells	Contain desmin.
Neuroglia	Contain glial fibrillary acidic proteins (GFAP).
Neurons	Contain neurofilaments.
Nucleus	Contains nuclear lamin.

Nissl bodies	Nissl bodies (in neurons) = rough ER; not found in axon or axon hillock. Synthesize enzymes (e.g., ChAT) and peptide neurotransmitters.	
Functions of Golgi apparatus	1. Distribution center of proteins and lipids from ER to the plasma membrane, lysosomes, and secretory vesicles 2. Modifies N-oligosaccharides 3. Adds O-oligosaccharides to serine and threonine residues 4. Proteoglycan assembly from proteoglycan core proteins 5. Sulfation of sugars in proteoglycans and of selected tyrosine on proteins 6. Addition of mannose-6-phosphate on specific lysosomal proteins, which targets the protein to the lysosome	I-cell disease is caused by the failure of addition of mannose-6-phosphate to lysosome proteins, causing these enzymes to be secreted outside the cell instead of being targeted to the lysosome.
Rough endoplasmic reticulum (RER)	Rough ER is the site of synthesis of secretory (exported) proteins and of N-linked oligosaccharide addition to many proteins.	Mucus-secreting goblet cells of the small intestine are rich in RER.

Smooth endoplasmic reticulum (SER) — Site of steroid synthesis and detoxification of drugs and poisons. | Liver hepatocytes and steroid-hormone-producing cells of the adrenal cortex are rich in SER.

Sinusoids of liver — Capillaries with round pores 100–200 nm in diameter without diaphragm. No basement membrane. Not a barrier to macromolecules of plasma (full access to surface of liver cells through space of Disse).

Sinusoids of spleen — Long, vascular channels in red pulp. With fenestrated "barrel hoop" basement membrane. Macrophages found nearby. | T cells are found in the PALS and the red pulp of the spleen. B cells are found in follicles within the white pulp of the spleen.

Pancreas endocrine cell types — Islets of Langerhans are collections of endocrine cells (most numerous in tail of pancreas). α = glucagon; β = insulin; δ = somatostatin. Islets arise from pancreatic buds.

Adrenal cortex zones
Zona **G**lomerulosa — Aldosterone (outer layer). | **GFR** corresponds with **s**alt (Na$^+$), **s**ugar (glucocorticoids), and **s**ex (androgens). "The deeper you go, the sweeter it gets."
Zona **F**asciculata — Cortisol (middle layer).
Zona **R**eticularis — Both cortisol and some androgens such as DHEA (inner layer).

Adrenal medulla — Chromaffin cells are only cells in the body that secrete epinephrine and norepinephrine. | Pheochromocytoma = most common tumor of the adrenal medulla in adults. Neuroblastoma = most common in children.

Types of secretion — Merocrine (eccrine) = by exocytosis (i.e., proteins). Apocrine = secretion with loss of cytoplasm from apical side (i.e., sweat). Holocrine = secretion with destruction of the cell (i.e., products of sebaceous glands). | *Apocrine* = *Apical* cytoplasm. *Holocrine* = *Whole* cytoplasm.

Brunner's glands — Secrete alkaline mucus. Located in submucosa of duodenum (the only GI submucosal glands). Duodenal ulcers cause hypertrophy of Brunner's glands. | **BAGS:** Brunner's Alkaline Glands, Submucosal.

Lymph node

A secondary lymphoid organ that has many afferents, one or more efferents. Encapsulated. With trabeculae. Functions are non-specific filtration by macrophages, storage/proliferation of B and T cells, Ab production.

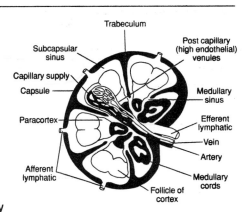

Follicle — Site of B-cell localization and proliferation. In outer cortex. 1° follicles are dense and dormant. 2° follicles have pale central germinal centers and are active.

Medulla — Consists of medullary cords (closely packed lymphocytes and plasma cells) and medullary sinuses. Medullary sinuses communicate with efferent lymphatics and contain reticular cells and macrophages.

Paracortex — Houses T cells. Region of cortex between follicles and medulla. Contains high endothelial venules into which T and B cells enter from blood. In an extreme cellular immune response, paracortex becomes greatly enlarged. Not well developed in patients with DiGeorge's syndrome.

Peyer's patch

Unencapsulated lymphoid tissue found in lamina propria and submucosa of intestine. Covered by single layer of cuboidal enterocytes (no goblet cells) with specialized M cells interspersed. M cells take up antigen.

IgA production in gut

Stimulated B cell leaves Peyer's patch and travels through lymph and blood to lamina propria of intestine. There, it differentiates to IgA-secreting plasma cell. IgA receives protective secretory piece, then is transported across epithelium to gut to deal with intraluminal Ag.

Think of **IgA**, the **I**ntra-**g**ut-**A**ntibody. And always say, "secretory IgA."

ANATOMY—NEUROANATOMY

Hypothalamus: functions

Thirst and water balance (supraoptic nucleus).
Adenohypophysis control via releasing factors.
Neurohypophysis control via direct neural impulses.
Hunger (lateral nucleus) and satiety (ventromedial nucleus).
Autonomic regulation, circadian rhythms (suprachiasmatic nucleus).
Temperature regulation:
  Post. hypothalamus—heat production when cold.
  Ant. hypothalamus—coordinates cooling when hot.
Sexual urges and emotions (septate nucleus).

The hypothalamus wears **"TAN HATS."**
If you zap your **P**osterior hypothalamus, you become a **P**oikilotherm (cold-blooded snake).
If you zap your ventromedial nucleus, you grow ventrally and medially (hyperphagia and obesity).

Posterior pituitary (neurohypophysis)

Receives hypothalamic projections from supraoptic (ADH) and paraventricular (oxytocin) nuclei.

Oxytocin: *oxys* = quick; *tocos* = birth.

Anotomy

HIGH-YIELD FACTS

Functions of thalamic nuclei	Lateral geniculate nucleus = visual. Medial geniculate nucleus = auditory. Ventral posterior nucleus, lateral part = proprioception, pressure, pain, touch vibration of body. Ventral posterior nucleus, medial part = facial sensation, including pain. Ventral anterior/lateral nuclei = motor.	
Limbic system: functions	Responsible for Feeding, Fighting, Feeling, Flight, and sex.	The famous 5 Fs.
CNS/PNS supportive cells	**A**strocytes—physical support, repair, K⁺ metabolism. **M**icroglia—phagocytosis. **O**ligodendroglia—central myelin production. **S**chwann cells—peripheral myelin production. **E**pendymal cells—inner lining of ventricles.	"**A MOSE** (like 'most') wonderful array of neural supportive cells."
Blood–brain barrier	Formed by three structures: 1. arachnoid 2. choroid plexus epithelium 3. intracerebral capillary endothelium Glucose and amino acids cross by carrier-mediated transport mechanism. Nonpolar/lipid-soluble substances cross more readily than polar/water-soluble ones.	Other barriers include: 1. blood–bile barrier 2. blood–testis barrier 3. blood–PNS barrier Example: L-dopa, rather than dopamine, is used to treat parkinsonism.
Chorea	Sudden, jerky, purposeless movements. Characteristic of basal ganglia lesion (e.g., Huntington's disease).	*Chorea* = dancing (Greek). Think choral dancing.
Athetosis	Slow, writhing movements, especially of fingers. Characteristic of basal ganglia lesion.	Think snakelike. *Athetos* = not fixed (Greek).
Hemiballismus	Sudden, wild flailing of one arm. Characteristic of subthalamic nucleus lesion.	Half ballistic (as in throwing a baseball).
Tremors: cerebellar versus basal	Cerebellar tremor = intention tremor. Basal ganglion tremor = resting tremor.	Basal = at rest.

Brain lesions

Area of lesion	Consequence
Broca's area	Motor (expressive) aphasia
Wernicke's area	Sensory (fluent) aphasia
Amygdala (bilateral)	Klüver-Bucy syndrome (hyperorality, hypersexuality, disinhibited behavior)
Frontal lobe	Frontal release signs (e.g., personality changes and deficits in concentration, orientation, judgment)
Right parietal lobe	Spacial neglect syndrome (agnosia of the contralateral side of the world)
Reticular activating system	Coma
Mamillary bodies (bilateral)	Korsakoff's syndrome (confabulations, anterograde amnesia)

BROca's is BROken speech.
Wernicke's is Wordy but makes no sense.

Cranial nerves

		Function	Type	
Olfactory	I	Smell	Sensory	Some
Optic	II	Sight	Sensory	Say
Oculomotor	III	Eye movement, pupil constriction, accommodation, eyelid opening	Motor	Marry
Trochlear	IV	Eye movement	Motor	Money
Trigeminal	V	Mastication, facial sensation	Both	But
Abducens	VI	Eye movement	Motor	My
Facial	VII	Facial movement, anterior 2/3 taste, lacrimation, salivation (submaxillary and submandibular salivary glands)	Both	Brother
Vestibulocochlear	VIII	Hearing, balance	Sensory	Says
Glossopharyngeal	IX	Posterior 1/3 taste, swallowing, salivation (parotid gland), monitoring carotid body and sinus	Both	Big
Vagus	X	Taste, swallowing, palate elevation, talking, thoracoabdominal viscera	Both	Brains
Accessory	XI	Head turning, shoulder shrugging, talking	Motor	Matter
Hypoglossal	XII	Tongue movements	Motor	Most

Cranial nerves and passageways

Cribriform plate	I
Optic canal	II
Superior orbital fissure	III, IV, V$_1$, VI
Foramen rotundum	V$_2$
Foramen ovale	V$_3$
Internal auditory meatus	VII, VIII
Jugular foramen	IX, X, XI
Hypoglossal canal	XII

Cavernous sinus

CN III, IV, V, VI all pass through the cavernous sinus. Only CN VI is "free-floating." Also contains cavernous portion of internal carotid artery.

The nerves that control extraocular muscles (plus V$_1$) pass through the cavernous sinus.

Foramina: middle cranial fossa	1. Optic canal (CN II, ophthalmic artery, central retinal vein) 2. Superior orbital fissure (CN III, IV, V_1, VI, ophthalmic vein) 3. Foramen **R**otundum (CN V_2) 4. Foramen **O**vale (CN V_3) 5. Foramen spinosum (middle meningeal artery) 6. Foramen lacerum (nothing really)	All structures pass through sphenoid bone. Divisions of CN V exit owing to **S**tanding **R**oom **O**nly (**S**uperior orbital fissure, foramen **R**otundum, foramen **O**vale).
Foramina: posterior cranial fossa	1. Internal auditory meatus (CN VII, VIII) 2. Jugular foramen (CN IX, X, XI, jugular vein) 3. Hypoglossal canal (CN XII) 4. Foramen magnum (spinal roots of CN XI, brain stem, vertebral arteries)	All structures pass through temporal or occipital bones.
Extraocular muscles and nerves	**L**ateral **R**ectus is CN VI, **S**uperior **O**blique is CN IV, rest are CN III.	The "chemical formula" LR_6SO_4, rest is CN III.
KLM sounds: kuh, la, mi	**K**uh-kuh-kuh tests palate elevation (CN X—vagus). **L**a-la-la tests tongue (CN XII—hypoglossal). **M**i-mi-mi tests lips (CN VII—facial).	Try it yourself.

Vagal nuclei
  Nucleus **s**olitarius
 	
  Nucleus **a**mbiguus
 	
  Dorsal motor nucleus
	
	Visceral **s**ensory information (e.g., taste, gut distention, etc.).
	Motor innervation of pharynx, larynx, and upper esophagus.
	Sends autonomic (mainly parasympathetic) fibers to heart, lungs, and upper GI.	

Lesions and deviations	CN XII lesion (LMN): tongue deviates **toward** side of lesion. CN V motor lesion: jaw deviates **toward** side of lesion. Unilateral lesion of cerebellum: patient tends to fall **toward** side of lesion.	
Dorsal column organization	In dorsal columns, lower limbs are inside to avoid crossing the upper limbs on the outside. Fasciculus gracilis = legs. Fasciculus cuneatus = arms.	Dorsal column is organized like you are, with hands at sides—arms outside and legs inside. *Gracilis* (Latin) = graceful, slender, like ballerina's legs.
Brown-Séquard syndrome	Lateral hemisection of spinal cord. Findings: 1. Ipsilateral motor paralysis and spasticity (pyramidal tract) 2. Ipsilateral tactile and motor loss (dorsal column lesion) 3. Contralateral pain and temperature loss (spinothalamic tract) 4. Minimal change in simple touch	

Lower motor neuron (LMN) signs	LMN injury signs: atrophy, flaccid paralysis, absent deep tendon reflexes. Fasciculations may be present.	**Lower** MN ≈ everything **lower**ed (less muscle mass, **decreased** muscle tone, **decreased** reflexes, **down**going toes).
Upper motor neuron (UMN) signs	UMN injury signs: little atrophy, spastic paralysis, hyperactive deep tendon reflexes, possible positive Babinski.	**Upper** MN ≈ everything **up** (tone, DTRs, toes).

Spindle muscle control

Reflex arc	Muscle spindle stretch stimulates Ia afferents. Ia stimulates alpha motor neurons of agonist muscle to contract extrafusal muscle fibers.
Gamma loop	Gamma motor neurons from CNS contract intrafusal muscle fibers → stretch spindle → reflex arc → stimulate alpha motor neuron. Responsible for maintaining tone.

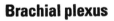

Visual field defects

1. Right anopsia
2. Bitemporal hemianopsia (tunnel vision)
3. Left homonymous hemianopsia
4. Left upper quadrantic anopsia (right temporal lesion)
5. Left lower quadrantic anopsia (right parietal lesion)

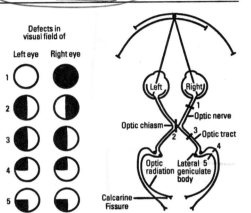

Brachial plexus

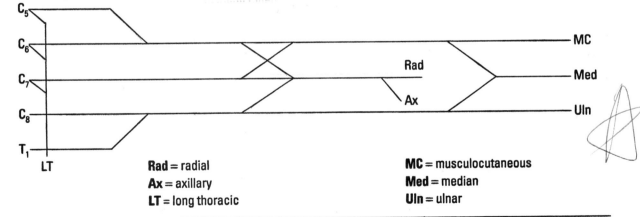

Rad = radial
Ax = axillary
LT = long thoracic

MC = musculocutaneous
Med = median
Uln = ulnar

Myotome "dances" (perform while reciting aloud)

Arm:
- **C5** —abduct arm
- **C678**—adduct arm
- **C56** —flex elbow
- **C78** —extend elbow
- **C6** —pronate/supinate
- **C67** —flex/extend wrist
- **C78** —flex/extend fingers
- **T1** —abduct/adduct fingers

Leg:
- **L123** —flex, adduct, medially rotate hip
- **L34** —extend knee
- **L45** —dorsiflex and invert ankle
- **L5,S1**—evert ankle
- **S12** —plantar flex

Cervical rib

An embryological defect; can compress subclavian artery and inferior trunk of brachial plexus (C8, T1), resulting in:

1. Atrophy of the thenar and hypothenar eminences
2. Atrophy of the interosseous muscles
3. Sensory deficits on the medial side of the forearm and hand
4. Disappearance of the radial pulse upon moving the head toward the opposite side

---

Facial lesion

Central facial

Paralysis of the contralateral facial muscles except the frontalis and orbicularis oculi muscles. Because the frontalis and orbicularis oculi muscles receive bilateral cortical innervation, they are not paralyzed by lesions involving one motor cortex or its corticobulbar pathways.

Bell's palsy

Peripheral facial paralysis.
Can occur idiopathically.
Seen as a complication in diabetes, tumors, sarcoidosis, AIDS, and Lyme disease.
Bell's phenomenon—when an attempt is made to close the eyelid, the eyeball on the affected side may turn upward.
Complete destruction of the facial nucleus itself or its branchial efferent fibers (facial nerve proper) paralyzes all ipsilateral facial muscles.

Embryology

1. Embryology of the heart, lung, kidney, and liver (i.e., what are the embryonic structures that give rise to these organs?).
2. Common embryological malformations (e.g., neural tube defects, cleft palate, tetralogy of Fallot, horseshoe kidney).
3. Embryological derivatives of the mesonephric (wolffian) and paramesonephric (müllerian) ducts and associated congenital abnormalities (e.g., testicular feminization).
4. Embryological derivatives of the fetal brain (e.g., telencephalon → cerebral hemispheres).
5. Embryological derivatives of the foregut, midgut, and hindgut.

Gross Anatomy

1. Anatomic landmarks in relation to medical procedures (e.g., thoracocentesis, lumbar puncture, pericardiocentesis).
2. Anatomical landmarks in relation to major organs (e.g., lungs, heart, kidneys).
3. Common injuries of the knee, hip, shoulder, and clavicle (e.g., shoulder separation, hip fracture).
4. Clinical features and anatomic correlations of specific brachial plexus lesions (e.g., waiter's tip, wrist drop, claw hand, scapular winging).
5. Clinical features of common peripheral nerve injuries (e.g., common peroneal nerve palsy, radial nerve palsy).
6. Etiology and clinical features of common diseases affecting the hands (e.g., carpal tunnel syndrome, cubital tunnel syndrome, Dupuytren's contracture).
7. Anatomy and physiology of blood-testis barrier.

Histology (Pexxen Wheater)

1. Histology of the respiratory tract structures (e.g., bronchi, respiratory bronchioles, and alveoli).
2. Function of pulmonary ciliary elevator.
3. Structure and function of endoplasmic reticulum and Golgi apparatus.
4. Structure and function of the mitochondrion.
5. Appearance of major cellular organelles and structures (e.g., ribosomes, mitochondria) on electron microscopy.
6. Structure and function of cell-cell junctions (e.g., tight junctions, desmosomes, gap junctions).
7. Histology of lymphoid organs (e.g., lymph nodes, thymus, spleen).
8. Phagocytic cells associated with different organ systems (e.g., Kupffer cells, alveolar macrophages, microglia, Langerhans cells).
9. Cellular biology of muscle contraction.
10. Histology and description of bone ossification (intermembranous vs. endochondral ossification), especially the growth plate.

Neuroanatomy

1. Etiology and clinical features of the brain, cranial nerve, and spinal cord disorders (e.g., Brown-Séquard syndrome).
2. Production, composition, and circulation of cerebrospinal fluid.

HIGH-YIELD FACTS

Anatomy

3. Neuroanatomy of hearing (central and peripheral hearing loss).
4. Structure and function of a chemical synapse (e.g., neuromuscular junction).
5. Major neurotransmitters (names, sites of production, excitatory versus inhibitory).
6. Mechanisms of neurotransmitter and hormone receptor function, including second messengers (e.g., norepinephrine, insulin, acetylcholine, GABA).
7. Blood supply of the brain (e.g., posterior cerebral artery) and neurological deficits corresponding to various vascular occlusions.
8. Functional anatomy of basal ganglia components (e.g., globus pallidus, amygdala).
9. Anatomical landmarks surrounding the pituitary gland.
10. Basic structural neuroanatomy as seen on CT and MR scans.

Behavioral Science

A heterogeneous mix of psychology, epidemiology/biostatistics, psychiatry, sociology, psychopharmacology, and more falls under this heading. Many medical students do not study this discipline diligently because the material is felt to be "easy" or "common sense." In our opinion, this is a missed opportunity. Each question gained in behavioral science is equal to a question in any other section in determining the overall score. At many medical schools, this material is not covered in a single course. Many students feel that some behavioral science questions are less concrete and require awareness of social aspects of medicine. Basic biostatistics and epidemiology are very learnable and thus high yield. Be able to apply biostatistical concepts such as specificity and predictive values in a problem-solving format.

Epidemiology
Ethics
Life Cycle
Physiology
Psychiatry
Psychology
High-Yield Topics

Behavioral Science

HIGH-YIELD FACTS

Prevalence versus incidence	Prevalence is total number of cases in a population at a given time. Incidence is number of new cases in a population per unit time; epidemic is when observed incidence greatly exceeds expected incidence.	Incidence is new incidents.
Sensitivity	Number of true positives divided by number of all people with the disease. False negative ratio is equal to **1** – sensitivity.	**PID** = **P**ositive **I**n **D**isease (note that PID is a sensitive topic).
Specificity	Number of true negatives divided by number of all people without the disease. False positive ratio is equal to **1** – specificity.	**NIH** = **N**egative **I**n **H**ealth.

Predictive value

Positive predictive value

Number of true positives divided by number of people who tested positive for the disease.

The probability of having a condition, given a positive test.

Negative predictive value

Number of true negatives divided by number of people who tested negative for the disease.

The probability of not having the condition, given a negative test.

Unlike sensitivity and specificity, predictive value is dependent on the prevalence of the disease.

The higher the prevalence of a disease, the higher the positive predictive value of the test.

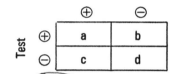

$$\text{Sensitivity} = \frac{a}{a+c}$$

$$\text{Specificity} = \frac{d}{b+d}$$

$$\text{PPV} = \frac{a}{a+b}$$

$$\text{NPV} = \frac{d}{c+d}$$

Odds ratio and relative risk

Odds ratio

Approximates the relative risk if the prevalence of the disease is not too high. Used for retrospective studies (e.g., case-control studies).

$$\text{OR} = ad / bc$$

Relative risk

Disease risk in exposed group/disease risk in unexposed group.

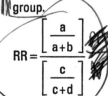

$$\text{RR} = \frac{\left[\dfrac{a}{a+b}\right]}{\left[\dfrac{c}{c+d}\right]} \qquad \text{Attributable Risk} = \left[\frac{a}{a+b}\right] - \left[\frac{c}{c+d}\right]$$

Standard deviation versus error	n = sample size, σ = standard deviation, SEM = standard error of the mean, SEM = $\sigma/\sqrt{n}$ Therefore, SEM < σ and SEM $\downarrow$ as $n \uparrow$.	If distribution is normal (Gaussian), then ± 1 σ contains 68% of values, ± 2 σ contains 95% of values, and ± 3 σ contains 99.7% of values.
Distribution: skew, bimodal	Terms that describe statistical distributions: Normal ≈ Gaussian ≈ bell-shaped. (Mean = median = mode.) Bimodal is simply two humps. Positive skew is asymmetry with tail on the right. Negative skew has tail on the left.	Positive skew = tail on more positive side (mean > median > mode). Negative skew = tail on more negative side (mean < median < mode).
Precision vs. accuracy	Precision is: 1. The consistency and reproducibility of a test (reliability) 2. The absence of random variation in a test. Accuracy is the trueness of test measurements.	Random error = reduced precision in a test. Systemic error = reduced accuracy in a test.
Reliability and validity	Reliability = reproducibility of a test; for example, inter-rater reliability (two examiners, statistic is called weighted κ) and split-half reliability (test on two equal groups). Dependability of a test. Validity = whether the test truly measures what it purports to measure. Appropriateness of a test.	Test is reliable if repeat measurements are the same. Test is valid if it measures what it is supposed to measure.
Correlation coefficient (r)	r is always between −1 and 1. Absolute value indicates strength of correlation. Pearson coefficient is used when values are evaluated directly. Spearman (rank) coefficient is used when values are placed in rank order and ranks are analyzed. Coefficient of determination = r^2.	**Spearmen** stand in ranks.
***t*-test versus ANOVA versus χ^2**	*t*-test checks difference between two means. ANOVA analyzes variance of three or more variables. χ^2 checks difference between two or more percentages or proportions of categorical outcomes (not mean values).	*t*-test = compare means. **ANOVA** = **AN**alysis **O**f **VA**riance of three or more variables. χ^2 = compare percentages (%) or proportions.
Confidence intervals	Standard 95% confidence interval is an interval that has a 95% probability of containing the true mean.	The smaller the interval, the more precise the estimate.
Meta-analysis	Pooling data from several studies to achieve greater statistical power.	Can't overcome limitations of individual studies or bias in study selection.

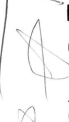

Behavioral Science · HIGH-YIELD FACTS

Case-control study

Observational study. Sample chosen based on presence (cases) or absence (controls) of disease. Information collected about risk factors.

Retrospective study.

Cohort study

Observational study. Sample chosen based on presence or absence of risk factors. Subjects followed over time for development of disease.

Prospective study.

Clinical trial

Experimental study. Compares therapeutic benefit of 2 or more treatments.

Highest-quality study.

Statistical hypotheses

Null (H_0)

Hypothesis of no difference (e.g., there is no association between the disease and the risk factor in the population).

Alternative (H_1)

Hypothesis that there is some difference (e.g., there is some association between the disease and the risk factor in the population).

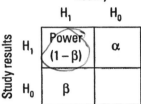

Reality

	H_1	H_0
H_1	Power $(1-\beta)$	α
H_0	β	

Study results

Type I error (α)

Stating that there is an effect or difference when there really is not (to mistakenly accept the experimental hypothesis and reject the null hypothesis). α is the probability of making a type I error and is equal to p (usually $< .05$).
p = probability of making a type I error.

If $p < .05$, then there is less than a 5% chance that the data will show something that is not really there. α = you "saw" a difference that did not exist— e.g., convicting an innocent man.

Type II error (β)

Stating that there **is not** an effect or difference when there really is (to fail to reject the null hypothesis when in fact H_0 is false). β is the probability of making a type II error.

β = you did not "see" a difference that does exist—e.g., setting a guilty man free.
$1 - \beta$ is "power" of study, or probability that study will see a difference if it is there.

Power

Probability of rejecting null hypothesis when it is in fact false. It depends on
1. Total number of end points experienced by population
2. Difference in compliance between treatment groups (differences in the mean values between groups)

If one increases sample size, one will increase power. There is power in numbers.
Power = $1 - \beta$.

Hollingshead determinants of socioeconomic status

The Hollingshead "3 factor" correlates are occupation, education, and residence. The "2 factor" correlates are occupation and education. Low SES associated with ↓ mental health, ↑ disabling disease, and ↑ smoking.

Premature infants	Defined as under 2500 g or 34 wk. Have greater physical and emotional problems. Complications of prematurity include low birth weight, infections, respiratory distress syndrome, necrotizing enterocolitis, and persistent fetal circulation.	
Fetal alcohol syndrome	Newborns of mothers who consumed significant amounts of alcohol during pregnancy have a higher incidence of congenital abnormalities, including pre- and postnatal developmental retardation, microcephaly, facial abnormalities, limb dislocation, heart and lung fistulas. Mechanism may include inhibition of cell migration.	
Apgar score (at birth)	Score 0–2 at 1 and 5 min in each of five categories: 1. Heart rate (0, <100, 100+) 2. Respiratory effort (0, irregular, regular) 3. Muscle tone (limp, some, active) 4. Reflex irritability (0, grimace, grimace + cough) 5. Color (blue/pale, trunk pink, all pink) 10 is perfect score.	**A** = appearance (color) **P** = pulse **G** = grimace **A** = activity **R** = respiration After Virginia Apgar, a famous neonatologist.
Heroin addiction	Approximately 500,000 US addicts. Heroin is schedule I (not prescribable). Evidence of addiction is narcotic abstinence syndrome (dilated pupils, lacrimation, rhinorrhea, sweating, yawning, irritability, and muscle aches). Also look for track marks (needle sticks in veins). Related diagnoses are hepatitis, abscesses, overdose, hemorrhoids, AIDS, right-sided endocarditis.	Naloxone (Narcan) and Naltrexone competitively inhibit opioids. Methadone (long-acting oral opiate) for heroin detoxification or long-term maintenance.
Reportable diseases	Only some infectious diseases are reported, including AIDS (but not HIV positivity), chicken pox, gonorrhea, hepatitis A and B, measles, mumps, rubella, salmonella, shigella, syphilis, tuberculosis.	

Leading causes of death in the US by age

Infants	Congenital anomalies, sudden infant death syndrome, short gestation/low birth weight, respiratory distress syndrome, maternal complications of pregnancy.	AIDS is leading cause of death in men between the ages of 20 and 40.
Age 1–14	Injuries, cancer, congenital anomalies, homicide, heart disease.	
Age 15–24	Injuries, homicide, suicide, cancer, heart disease.	
Age 25–64	Cancer, heart disease, injuries, stroke, suicide.	
Age 65+	Heart disease, cancer, stroke, COPD, pneumonia.	

Elderly population in year 2000	In year 2000, estimated US population = 300,000,000. 35 million > 65 y old. Greatest increase in those > 85 y old.	13% of US population > 65 y old in year 2000.
Risk factors for suicide completion	White, male, alone, prior attempts, presence and lethality of plan, medical illness, alcohol or drug use, on 3 or more prescription medications.	

Common surgeries	Dilation and curettage, hysterectomy, tonsillectomy, sterilization, hernia, oophorectomy, cesarean section, cholecystectomy.	Mostly done on women.
Divorce statistics	US has highest rate. Teenage marriages at high risk. More common when religions are mixed. Peaks at second/third year of marriage. Higher with low SES. Unrelated to industrialization. Divorcees remarry very frequently.	
Drug agencies	FDA = Food and Drug Administration (safety and efficacy of drugs). DEA = Drug Enforcement Administration (security of controlled substances). NIDA = National Institute on Drug Abuse (education, prevention).	FDA = protection. DEA = prosecution. NIDA = prevention.
Medicare, Medicaid	Medicare and Medicaid are federal programs that originated from amendments to the Social Security Act. Medicare Part A = hospital, Part B = supplemental. Medicaid is federal and state assistance for those on welfare or indigent.	**Medicare** is **care** for the elderly. **Medicaid** is **aid** for the poor. Medi-**Cal** is the **Cali**fornia version of Medicaid.

BEHAVIORAL SCIENCE—ETHICS

Futility
 	
	If medical situation is futile, physician may refuse patient's or family's request for intervention or may spare the patient an invasive intervention.
	Strict futility defined:
	   1. Intervention does not make sense pathophysiologically
	   2. Maximal treatment is failing
	   3. The intervention has already failed the patient
	   4. Intervention will not achieve the goals of care

Informed consent	Legally requires:
	   1. Discussion of pertinent information
	   2. Obtaining the patient's agreement to the plan of care
	   3. Freedom from coercion
		Patients must understand the risks, benefits and alternatives, including no intervention.

Exceptions to informed consent	**1.** Patient lacks decision-making capacity **2.** Implied consent in an emergency **3.** Therapeutic privilege—withholding information when disclosure would severely harm the patient or undermine informed decision-making capacity **4.** Waiver—patient waives the right of informed consent

Decision making capacity	1. Patient makes and communicates a choice 2. Patient is informed 3. Decision is stable over time 4. Decisions consistent with patient's values and goals 5. Decisions not a result of delusions or hallucinations
Advance directives	If medical situation is not futile but the patient is not capable of making an informed decision, is there an advance directive outlining the patient's wishes? If an advance directive does not exist, a physician may appoint and work with a surrogate decision maker.
Oral advance directive	Incapacitated patient's prior oral statements commonly used as guide. Problems arise from variance in interpretation of these statements. However, if patient was informed, directive is specific, patient makes a choice, and decision is repeated over time, the oral directive is more valid.
Written advance directive	1. Living wills—Patient directs physician to withhold or withdraw life-sustaining treatment if s/he develops a terminal disease or persistent vegetative state 2. Durable power of attorney—Patient designates a surrogate to make medical decisions in the event that s/he loses decision-making capacity. Patient may also specify decisions in clinical situations. More flexible than a living will.
Nonmaleficence	"Do no harm." However, if benefits of an intervention outweigh the risks, a patient may make an informed decision to proceed.
Beneficence	Physicians have a special ethical responsibility to act in the patient's best interest (physician is a fiduciary). Patient autonomy may conflict with beneficence. If the patient makes an informed decision, the patient ultimately has the right to decide.
Confidentiality	Confidentiality respects patient privacy and autonomy. Disclosing information to family and friends should be guided by what the patient would want. The patient may also waive the right to confidentiality (e.g., insurance companies).
Exceptions to confidentiality	1. Potential harm to third parties is serious 2. Likelihood of harm is high 3. No alternative means exist to warn or protect those at risk 4. Third party can take steps to prevent harm Once confidence breached, resulting harms are minimized and considered acceptable. Examples include: 1. Infectious diseases—physicians may have a duty to warn public officials and identifiable people at risk 2. The Tarasoff decision—law requiring physician to protect potential victim from harm; may involve breach of confidentiality 3. Child and elder abuse 4. Impaired automobile drivers 5. Suicidal/homicidal patient 6. Domestic violence (in California)

BEHAVIORAL SCIENCE—ETHICS (*continued*)

Malpractice

Civil suit under negligence requires
1. Physician breach of duty to patient
2. Patient suffers harm
3. Breach of duty causes harm

The **4 D's: D**ereliction of **D**uty
Directly led to **D**amage

BEHAVIORAL SCIENCE—LIFE CYCLE

Anaclitic depression

Anaclitic depression = depression in an infant owing to separation from household of caregiver. Can result in failure to thrive. Infant becomes withdrawn and unresponsive.

Ana = against; *clitic* = lean.

Regression in children

Children will regress to younger behavior under stress: physical illness, punishment, birth of a new sibling, tiredness. An example is bedwetting in a child when he is hospitalized.

Infant deprivation effects

Long-term deprivation of affection results in:
1. Decreased muscle tone
2. Poor language skills
3. Poor socialization skills
4. Lack of basic trust
5. Anaclitic depression
Severe deprivation can result in infant death.

Studied by René Spitz. The **4 Ws: W**eak, **W**ordless, **W**anting (socially), **W**ary. Deprivation for longer than 6 months can lead to irreversible changes.

Infancy stages

Normal autistic stage: 0–2 mo.
Normal symbiotic stage: 2–8 mo.
Separation/individuation stage: 9–18 mo.
Object constancy: 18–36 mo.

Described by Margaret Mahler.

Jean Piaget stages

Cognitive stages (intellectual development):
0–2 y: **S**ensorimotor
2–7 y: **P**reoperational (egocentric thinking)
7–11 y: **C**oncrete operational (conservation of volume)
11+ y: **F**ormal operational (abstract concepts)

Slowly, **P**iaget's **C**hildren **F**orm.

Erik Erikson stages

Stages of psychological development in which individual is confronted with major "tasks":
0–1 y: trust versus mistrust
1–3 y: autonomy versus shame/doubt
3–6 y: initiative versus guilt
6–12 y: industry versus inferiority
12–20 y: identity versus role confusion
20–30 y: intimacy versus isolation
30–65 y: generativity versus self-absorption
65+ y: ego integrity versus despair

Cutoff years are 1, 3, 6, 12, 20, 30, 65 (≈doubling).

Kübler-Ross dying stages	Denial, Anger, Bargaining, Grieving, Acceptance. Pathologic grief is grieving for >2 y, or overwhelmingly intense grief.	Death Arrives Bringing Grave Adjustments.
Memory loss with age	Generally, as you grow older you lose recent memory first, distant or remote memory last.	Old people tell great stories about the old days.

Endorphins and enkephalins	Both have opiate-like activities, are blocked by naloxone, lose activity over time. Enkephalins are pentapeptides (small). β-endorphin (31 amino acids) is derived from POMC.	Endorphin = **end**ogenous **morphine**. Also, Morpheus was the god of sleep.
Neurotransmitter changes with disease	Depression—decreased NE and serotonin (5-HT). Alzheimer's dementia—decreased ACh. Huntington's disease—decreased GABA, decreased ACh. Bipolar affective disorder—decreased serotonin (5-HT). Schizophrenia—increased dopamine. Parkinson's disease—decreased dopamine.	
Frontal lobe functions	Concentration, Orientation, Language, Abstraction, Judgment, Motor regulation, Mood. Lack of social judgment is most notable in frontal lobe lesion.	**COLA-JMM**
Hypothalamic nuclei		
Satiety	Ventromedial nucleus of hypothalamus controls appetite.	Ablating **ventromedial** nucleus will cause you to grow **ventr**ally and **medial**ly (you get fat).
Hunger	Lateral nucleus of hypothalamus.	

Sleep stages

	Description	Waveform
0—eyes open	Awake, alert, active mental concentration	Beta (highest frequency, lowest amplitude)
0—eyes closed	Awake	Alpha
1 (5%)	Light sleep	Theta
2 (45%)	Deeper sleep	Sleep spindles and K-complexes
3–4 (25%)	Deepest, non-REM sleep; sleepwalking; night terrors, bedwetting (slow-wave sleep)	Delta (lowest frequency, highest amplitude)
REM (25%)	Dreaming, loss of motor tone, possibly memory processing function, erections, ↑ brain O_2 use	Beta

1. Serotonergic predominance of raphe nucleus key to initiating sleep
2. Norepinephrine reduces REM sleep
3. Extraocular movements during REM due to activity of PPRF (parapontine reticular formation/conjugate gaze center)
4. REM sleep having the same EEG pattern as while awake and alert has spawned the terms "paradoxical sleep" and "desynchronized sleep"
5. Benzodiazepines shorten stage 4 sleep; thus useful for night terrors and sleepwalking
6. Imipramine is used to treat enuresis since it decreases stage 4 sleep

REM sleep

25% of total sleep. Occurs every 90 minutes; duration increases through the night. REM sleep decreases with age. Acetylcholine is the principal neurotransmitter involved in REM sleep.

REM rebound

Body compensates for any missed REM sleep. Drugs that decrease the amount of REM sleep (e.g., barbiturates, alcohol, phenothiazines, and MAO inhibitors) cause an increased amount of REM sleep after the specific drug is discontinued.

Benzodiazepines decrease the amount of REM sleep without causing REM rebound.

Sleep patterns of depressed patients

Patients with depression typically have the following changes in their sleep stages:
1. Reduced slow-wave sleep
2. Decreased REM latency
3. Early-morning waking

Sensory deprivation effects

1. Suppression of EEG
2. Decreased galvanic skin response
3. Decreased respiration
4. Increased urinary epinephrine

Seen in the ICU setting or after excessive studying.

Stress effects

Stress induces production of free fatty acids, 17-OH corticosteroids, lipids, cholesterol, catecholamines; affects water absorption, muscular tonicity, gastrocolic reflex, mucosal circulation.

Forensic psychiatry	Confidentiality: breachable in child abuse, emergencies, communicable diseases. Good samaritan law protects roadside MD from malpractice liability. Involuntary hold: danger to self, others, unable to provide food/clothing/shelter.	
Cultural/ethnic psychiatry	Specific diseases: Amok = killing rampage (seen in southeast Asia). Latah = echolalia, coprolalia (Malaysia). Koro = fear of penile regression, death (seen in Chinese men).	The origin of "running amok." Echolalia = repetition of another person's words or phrases. Coprolalia = "filthy" language.
Orientation as to person	Is the patient aware of himself as a person? Does he know his name? Anosognosia = unaware that one is ill. Autopagnosia = unable to locate one's own body parts. Depersonalization = body seems unreal or dissociated.	Generally, the last thing to go (first = time, second = place, last = person).
Orientation as to place	Deficiency in orientation as to place, including jamais vu (person is in a familiar surrounding but feels he or she has never been there before) and déjà vu (person is in an unfamiliar situation and feels he or she has been there before).	
Amnesia types	Anterograde amnesia is being unable to remember things that occurred after a CNS insult (no new memory). Korsakoff's amnesia is a classic anterograde amnesia that is caused by thiamine deficiency (bilateral destruction of the mamillary bodies), is seen in alcoholics, and is associated with confabulations. Retrograde amnesia is being unable to remember things that occurred before a CNS insult.	*Antero* = after; *retro* = before.
Substance dependence	Maladaptive pattern of substance use. Defined as 3 or more of the following signs in 1 year: 1. Tolerance 2. Withdrawal 3. Substance taken in larger amounts than intended 4. Persistent desire or attempts to cut down 5. Lots of energy spent trying to obtain substance 6. Important social, occupational or recreational activities given up or reduced because of substance use 7. Use continued despite knowing the problems that it causes	
Substance abuse	Maladaptive pattern leading to clinically significant impairment or distress. Symptoms have not met criteria for substance dependence. One or more of the following in 1 year: 1. Recurrent use resulting in failure to fulfill major obligations at work, school, or home 2. Recurrent use in physically hazardous situations 3. Recurrent substance-related legal problems 4. Continued use despite persistent problems caused by use	

HIGH-YIELD FACTS

Behavioral Science

Behavioral Science

HIGH-YIELD FACTS

Delirium	Decreased attention span and level of arousal, disorganized thinking, hallucination, illusions, misperceptions, disturbance in sleep-wake cycle, cognitive dysfunction. Key to diagnosis: waxing and waning level of consciousness, develops rapidly.	Delirium = changes in sensorium
Dementia	Development of multiple cognitive deficits: memory, aphasia, apraxia, agnosia, loss of abstract thought, behavioral/personality changes, impaired judgment. Key to diagnosis: rule out delirium—patient is alert, no change in level of consciousness. More often gradual onset.	Dememtia characterized by memory loss

Major depressive episode	Characterized by 5 of the following for 2 weeks including (1) depressed mood or (2) anhedonia:
	  1. Depressed mood by self-report or by observation
	  2. Marked decrease in interest/pleasure in activities most of the day
	  3. Weight changes (not dieting), or appetite changes
	  4. Sleep changes
	  5. Psychomotor agitation or retardation
	  6. Fatigue or loss of energy
	  7. Feelings of worthlessness or guilt
	  8. Decreased ability to concentrate or think
	  9. Recurrent thoughts of death
	Major depressive disorder, recurrent—requires 2 or more episodes with interval of 2 months where patient does not meet criteria.	

Manic episode	Distinct period of abnormally and persistently elevated, expansive or irritable mood lasting at least 1 week. During mood disturbance, 3 or more of the following:
	  1. Inflated self-esteem or grandiosity
	  2. Decreased need for sleep
	  3. Pressured speech
	  4. Flight of ideas or racing thoughts
	  5. Distractibility
	  6. Increase in goal-directed activity or psychomotor agitation
	  7. Excessive involvement in pleasurable activities that have a high potential for painful consequences	

Hypomanic episode	Like manic episode except mood disturbance not severe enough to cause marked impairment in social, occupational functioning or to necessitate hospitalization, and there are no psychotic features.	
Bipolar disorder	Six separate criteria sets exist for bipolar I disorders with combinations of manic, hypomanic, and depressed episodes.	
Cyclothymic disorder	For at least 2 years, period with hypomanic symptoms and depressed symptoms that do not meet criteria for major depressive episode.	

Malingering	Patient fakes or claims to have a disorder in order to attain a specific gain (e.g., financial).
Factitious disorder	Consciously creates symptoms but doesn't know why. Also known as Munchausen syndrome.
Somatoform disorders	Several types: 1. Conversion—symptoms suggest neurologic or physical disorder but tests and physical exam are negative 2. Somatoform pain disorder—conversion disorder with pain as presenting complaint 3. Hypochondriasis—misinterpretation of normal physical findings, leading to preoccupation with and fear of having a serious illness despite medical reassurance 4. Somatization—variety of complaints in multiple organ systems 5. Body dysmorphic disorder—patient convinced that part of own anatomy is malformed 6. Somatization in groups—groups of people share conversion disorder 7. Pseudocyesis—false belief of being pregnant associated with objective signs of pregnancy

Panic disorder

Discrete periods of intense fear or discomfort peaking in 10 minutes with 4 of the following:

1. Palpitations, racing heart	8. Dizziness, faintness, lightheadedness
2. Sweating	9. Derealization
3. Trembling	10. Fear of losing control
4. Shortness of breath	11. Fear of dying
5. Choking feeling	12. Paresthesias
6. Chest pain/discomfort	13. Chills or hot flashes
7. Nausea/abdominal distress	

Pain disorder must be diagnosed in context of occurrence (e.g., panic disorder with agoraphobia).

Specific phobia	Fear that is excessive or unreasonable, cued by presence or anticipation of a specific object or animal. Exposure provokes anxiety response. Person (not necessarily children) recognizes fear is excessive. Fear interferes with normal routine.
Social phobia	Fear of one or more social performance situations. Person fears acting in a way that is embarrassing or humiliating.
Obsession	Recurrent, intrusive and persistent thoughts, impulses or images that cannot be ignored or suppressed by logical effort. Associated with anxiety.
Compulsion	Repetitive behaviors or mental acts that person feels driven to perform. Committing act produces transient relief from anxiety.
Obsessive-compulsive disorder	Person realizes that either obsession or compulsion is excessive and is causing marked distress or interfering with normal routine. Person may have poor insight.

Post-traumatic stress disorder	Person experienced or witnessed event that involved actual or threatened death or serious injury. Response involves intense fear, helplessness, or horror. Traumatic event is persistently reexperienced, and person persistently avoids stimuli associated with the trauma. Person experiences persistent symptoms of increased arousal. Disturbance lasts longer than 1 month and causes distress or social/occupational impairment.	
Personality disorders	Personality trait is an enduring pattern of perceiving, relating to, and thinking about the environment and oneself that is exhibited in a wide range of important social and personal contexts. Personality disorder—when these patterns become inflexible and maladaptive causing impairment in social or occupational functioning or subjective distress.	
Cluster A personality disorder	Paranoid, schizoid, schizotypal: Characteristics: paranoid, suspicious, social isolation, odd beliefs, shy, withdrawn, impoverished personal relationships. Clinical dilemma: patient is suspicious of doctor and does not trust doctor.	
Cluster B personality disorder	Borderline, histrionic, narcissistic, antisocial Characteristics: dramatic, self-indulgent, hostile, aggressive, exploitative relationships, attention seeking. Clinical dilemma: patient will change rules on doctor. Clingy and demands attention. Feels that s/he is VIP and special. Will manipulate doctor.	
Cluster C personality disorder	Obsessive-compulsive, avoidant, dependent, passive aggressive Characteristics: fear of doing wrong thing, anxiety repressed, regulations, unable to express affect. Clinical dilemma: patient may subtly sabotage his/her own treatment. Person is very controlling.	
Narcolepsy	Dissociation of REM from sleep, resulting in hypnagogic (just before sleep) hallucinations and cataplexy (sudden loss of motor tone while awake). Associated with the appearance of REM sleep that occurs a few minutes after falling asleep. Strong genetic component.	Very accident prone. Treatment: stimulant drugs (e.g., amphetamines)
Hallucination versus illusion versus delusion	Hallucinations are perceptions in the absence of external stimuli. Illusions are misinterpretations of actual external stimuli. Delusions are false beliefs not shared with other members of culture/subculture that are firmly maintained in spite of obvious proof to the contrary.	
Delusion vs. loose association	A delusion is a disorder in the content of thought. A loose association is a disorder in the form of thought.	

Hallucination types	Visual hallucination is common in acute organic brain syndrome. Auditory hallucination is common in schizophrenia. Olfactory hallucination often occurs as an aura of a psychomotor epilepsy. Gustatory hallucination is rare. Tactile hallucination (e.g., formications) is common in delirium tremens. Also seen in cocaine abusers ("cocaine bugs"). Hypnagogic hallucination occurs while going to sleep. Hypnopompic hallucination occurs while waking from sleep.	

Schizophrenia	Waxing and waning vulnerability to psychosis (impaired reality testing, disordered behavior, thought disturbance), paranoia, delusions, auditory/visual hallucinations and disturbed affect.	

The **4 As** described by Bleuler:
1. **A**mbivalence (uncertainty)
2. **A**utism (self-preoccupation and lack of communication)
3. **A**ffect (blunted)
4. **A**ssociations (loose)

Fifth A should be **A**uditory hallucinations.
Genetic factors outweigh environmental factors in the etiology of schizophrenia.
Lifetime prevalence = 1.5% (males = females, blacks = whites).

Five subtypes:
1. Disorganized
2. Catatonic
3. Paranoid
4. Undifferentiated
5. Residual

Schneiderian signs of psychosis	1. Auditory hallucination 2. Thought broadcasting 3. Delusional perception 4. Experience of influence or alienation	

Antipsychotic mechanism	Antipsychotics most commonly work by blocking dopamine (D_2) receptors. Examples: haloperidol, chlorpromazine, thiothixene.	They stop a person from being a psychotic **dope** by blocking **dope**amine receptors.

Phobias	Over 100, so use etymology to figure them out. Examples include: Gamophobia (*gam* = gamete) = fear of marriage. Algophobia (*alg* = pain) = fear of pain. Acrophobia (*acro* = height) = fear of heights. Agoraphobia (*agora* = assembly) = fear of open places.	Systematic desensitization is a treatment used for phobias.

Projective tests	Projective tests use ambiguous stimuli. Examples: Rorschach (ink blot), TAT, sentence completion, word association, draw-a-person.	The patient projects his or her personality into the test.

Gain: 1°, 2°, 3°	1° gain = what the symptom does for the patient's internal psychic economy. 2° gain = what the symptom gets the patient (sympathy, attention). 3° gain = what the caretaker gets (like an MD on an interesting case).	

Behavioral Science

HIGH-YIELD FACTS

Electroconvulsive therapy	Occasional treatment of choice for major depression. ECT is painless, produces a seizure with transient memory loss and disorientation. Complications can result from anesthesia. The major adverse effect of ECT is retrograde amnesia.	Very controversial. Illegal in California as the first therapeutic modality.

Id, ego, superego	The structural hypothesis in psychoanalysis: Id = primal urges, sex, and aggression. (I want it.) Superego = conscience. (You know you can't have it.) Ego = mediator in id-superego conflicts. (I'll figure out how to cope with the conflict.)
Ego defenses	Think of all your ego defenses applied to studying: automatic, unconscious.
Acting out	Engaging in activities in a different area from the one in which the basic impulses come into conflict with values (e.g., vandalism).
Denial	Avoidance of awareness of some painful reality. A common reaction in newly diagnosed AIDS and cancer patients.
Displacement	Process whereby avoided ideas and feelings are transferred to some other person, situation, or object. Seen in phobias.
Doing and undoing	Expression of both an impulse and its opposite, usually in rapid succession.
Fixation	Partially remaining at a more childish level of development.
Identification	Becoming more like someone else.
Isolation	Splitting of ideas and feelings.
Projection	An unacceptable internal impulse or idea is attributed to an external source (e.g., other people). Common in paranoid states.
Rationalization	Proclaiming logical reasons for actions actually performed for other reasons, usually to avoid stress of self-blame.
Reaction formation	Process whereby a warded-off idea or feeling is replaced by an unconsciously derived but consciously felt emphasis on its opposite.
Regression	Turning back the maturational clock and going back to earlier modes of dealing with the world (a common reaction to hospitalization). Seen in children under stress (e.g., bedwetting) and in patients on peritoneal dialysis.
Repression	Involuntary withholding from conscious awareness an idea or feeling.
Sublimation	Process whereby one replaces an unacceptable wish with a course of action that is similar to the wish but does not conflict with one's value system.
Suppression	Voluntary (unlike other defenses) withholding of an idea or feeling from conscious awareness.
Dissociation	Seen in patients with multiple personality disorder.
Sick role	Exempts sick person from duties, allows person to expect care and condolences, and obligates sick person to try to get well (i.e., working toward being healthy, cooperation with health care personnel in getting well, and compliance with the treatment regimen).

Dyad	A pair of people within an interactional situation (e.g., husband-wife, mother-child, therapist-patient).	
Factors in hopelessness	Four dynamic factors in the development of hopelessness: 1. Sense of **I**mpotence (powerlessness) 2. Sense of **G**uilt 3. Sense of **A**nger 4. Sense of loss/**D**eprivation leading to depression	**IGAD!**
Conditioners: fear	Moderate fear is better than severe or mild fear in changing behavior.	As in studying for big exams.
Conditioning: classical	Learning in which a response is elicited by an unconditioned stimulus alone that previously was presented in conjunction with the conditioned stimulus, e.g., disulfiram (Antabuse) therapy in alcoholics.	Programmed by habit, without any element of reward. As in Pavlov's **classical** experiments with dogs (ringing the bell provoked salivation).
Conditioning: operant	Learning in which a particular action is elicited because it produces a reward.	Voluntary action and a reward.

Reinforcement schedules

Continuous Variable ratio	Shows the most rapid extinction when discontinued. Shows the slowest extinction when discontinued.	This explains why people can get addicted to slot machines at casinos and yet get upset when vending machines don't work.
Gestalt therapy	Stresses treatment of the whole person, highlights sensory awareness of the here and now, uses role playing. Developed by Frederick Perls.	
Psychoanalysis	A form of insight therapy—intensive, lengthy, costly, great demands on patient, developed by Freud. May be appropriate for changing chronic character problems.	
Topography (in psychoanalysis)	Conscious = what you are aware of. Preconscious = what you are able to make conscious with effort (like your phone number). Unconscious = what you are not aware of; the central goal of Freudian psychotherapy is to make the patient aware of what is hidden in his/her unconscious.	
Existential psychotherapy	Emphasis on confrontation and feeling experiences; each individual is responsible for his or her own existence.	
Intelligence testing	Stanford-Binet and Wechsler are the most famous tests. Mean is defined at 100, with standard deviation of 15. IQ less than 70 (or 2 standard deviations below the mean) is one of the criteria for diagnosis of mental retardation. IQ scores are correlated with genetic factors, but are more highly correlated with school achievement.	

Sexual dysfunction	Differential diagnosis includes:
	1. Drugs (e.g., antihypertensives, neuroleptics, ethanol)
	2. Diseases (e.g., depression, diabetes)
	3. Psychological (e.g., performance anxiety)

Changes in the elderly	As one gets older:
	1. Suicide rate increases
	2. Psychological problems (e.g., depression) become more prevalent
	3. Ejaculation takes longer to reach
	4. In females, vaginal barrel length and vaginal lubrication decrease

Epidemiology/Biostatistics

1. Differences in the incidence of disease among various ethnic groups.
2. Leading causes and types of cancers in men versus women.
3. Prevalence of common psychiatric disorders (e.g., alcoholism, major depression, schizophrenia).
4. Differences in death rates among ethnic and racial groups.
5. Definitions of morbidity, mortality, and case fatality rate.
6. Epidemiology of cigarette smoking, including prevalence and success rates for quitting.
7. Modes of human immunodeficiency virus (HIV) transmission among different populations (e.g., perinatal, heterosexual, homosexual, intravenous).
8. Simple pedigree analysis for inheritance of genetic diseases (e.g., counseling, risk assessment).
9. Different types of studies (e.g., randomized clinical trial, cohort, case series).
10. Definition and use of standard deviation, p value, r value, mean, mode, and median.

Neurophysiology

1. Physiologic changes (e.g., neurotransmitter levels) in common neuropsychiatric disorders (e.g., Alzheimer's disease, Huntington's disease, schizophrenia, bipolar disorder).
2. Changes in cerebrospinal fluid composition with common psychiatric diseases (e.g., depression).
3. Physiological, physical, and psychological changes associated with aging (e.g., memory, lung capacity, glomerular filtration rate, muscle mass, pharmacokinetics of drugs).
4. Differences between anterior and posterior lobes of the pituitary gland (e.g., embryology, innervation, hormones).

Psychiatry/Psychology

1. Diagnosis of common psychiatric disorders.
2. Indicators of prognosis in psychiatric disorders (e.g., schizophrenia, bipolar disorder).
3. Genetic components of common psychiatric disorders (e.g., schizophrenia, bipolar disorder).
4. Diseases associated with different personality types.
5. Clinical features and treatment of phobias.
6. Clinical features of child abuse.
7. Clinical features of common learning disorders (e.g., dyslexia, mental retardation).
8. Therapeutic application of learning theories (e.g., classical and operant conditioning) to psychiatric illnesses (e.g., disulfiram therapy for alcoholics).
9. Problems associated with the physician-patient relationship (e.g., reasons for patient noncompliance).
10. Management of the suicidal patient.

Biochemistry

This high-yield material includes cofactors, vitamins, essential minerals, genetic diseases involving single-enzyme deficiencies, general principles of metabolism, and cell and molecular biology. The first four topics are especially high yield and are worth learning in detail. There is little emphasis on hardcore organic chemistry, mechanisms, and physical chemistry. Don't emphasize this difficult material if you don't already know it. Detailed chemical structures are infrequently tested. Familiarity with the latest biochemical techniques that have medical relevance—such as enzyme-linked immunosorbent assay, immunoelectrophoresis, Southern blotting, and PCR—is useful. Beware if you placed out of your medical school's biochemistry class, for the emphasis of the test differs from the emphasis of many undergraduate courses.

DNA and RNA
Genetic Errors
Metabolism
Protein/Cell
Vitamins
High-Yield Topics

Biochemistry

HIGH-YIELD FACTS

Chromatin structure

Condensed by (−) charged DNA looped twice around (+) charged H2A, H2B, H3, and H4 histones (nucleosome bead). H1 ties nucleosomes together in a string (30-nm fiber). In mitosis DNA condenses to form mitotic chromosomes.

Think of beads on a string.

Heterochromatin — Condensed, transcriptionally inactive.

Euchromatin — Less condensed, transcriptionally active.

Eu = true, "truly transcribed."

Nucleotides

Purines (A, G) have two rings. Pyrimidines (C, T, U) have one ring. Guanine has a ketone. Thymine has a methyl.

CUT the PY (pie): pyrimidines
PURe As Gold: purines
THYmine has a meTHYl

AUG codon

AUG (or rarely GUG) is the mRNA initiation codon. AUG codes for methionine, which may be removed before translation is completed. In prokaryotes the initial AUG codes for a formyl-methionine (f-met).

AUG in**AUG**urates protein synthesis.

Genetic code: features

Unambiguous = each codon specifies only one amino acid.
Degenerate = more than one codon may code for same amino acid.
Commaless, nonoverlapping (except some viruses).
Universal (exceptions include mitochondria, archaebacteria, *Mycoplasma,* and some yeasts).

Mutations in DNA

Silent = same aa, often base change in third position of codon.
Missense = changed aa. (Conservative = new aa is similar in chemical structure.)
Nonsense = change resulting in early stop codon.

Severity of damage: nonsense > missense > silent.

Transition versus transversion

Transition = substituting purine for purine or pyrimidine for pyrimidine.
Transversion = substituting purine for pyrimidine or vice versa.

Transversion = **Trans**conversion (one type to another).

DNA replication	Multiple origins of replication: continuous DNA synthesis on leading strand and discontinuous (Okazaki fragments) on lagging strand. DNA polymerase reaches primer of preceding fragment; 5′ → 3′ exonuclease activity of DNA polymerase degrades RNA; DNA ligase seals; 3′ → 5′ exonuclease activity of DNA polymerase "proofreads" each added nucleotide.	Eukaryotic genome has multiple origins of replication. Bacteria, viruses and plasmids have only one origin of replication
Polymerases: DNA	Functions in *E. coli*: DNA polymerase I removes RNA primers, fills gaps, and participates in repair. DNA polymerase II function is unknown. DNA polymerase III (holoenzyme) elongates most efficiently, makes bulk of DNA (high fidelity).	Enzymes that proofread cannot initiate (because initiation is a sloppy process). **Primase makes an RNA primer on which DNA polymerase can initiate replication.**
Polymerase chain reaction (PCR)	Molecular biology laboratory procedure that is used to synthesize many copies of a desired fragment of DNA. Steps: 1. DNA strands are separated by heating 2. During cooling, excess of pre-made primer binds to the DNA sequence to be amplified 3. Heat-stable DNA polymerase replicates the DNA These steps are repeated multiple times for DNA sequence amplification.	
DNA repair: single strand	Single-strand, excision-repair-specific glycosylase recognizes and removes damaged base. Endonuclease makes a break several bases to the 5′ side. Exonuclease removes short stretch of nucleotides. DNA polymerase fills gap. DNA ligase seals.	If both strands are damaged, repair may proceed via recombination with undamaged homologous chromosome.
DNA/RNA synthesis direction	DNA and RNA are both synthesized 5′ → 3′. Remember that the 5′ of the incoming nucleotide bears the triphosphate (energy source for bond). The 3′ hydroxyl of the nascent chain is the target.	Imagine the incoming nucleotide bringing a gift (triphosphate) to the 3′ host. **BYOP (phosphate) from 5 to 3.**
Polymerases: RNA	**Eukaryotes:** RNA polymerase I makes rRNA. RNA polymerase II makes mRNA. RNA polymerase III makes tRNA. No proofreading function, but can initiate chains. RNA polymerase II opens DNA at promoter site (A-T-rich upstream sequence—TATA and CAAT). α-amanitin inhibits RNA polymerase II. **Prokaryotes:** RNA polymerase makes all three kinds of RNA.	I, II, and III are numbered as their products are used in protein synthesis. Or I, II, III ≈ ReMoTe.

Introns versus exons	Exons contain the actual genetic information coding for protein. Introns are intervening noncoding segments of DNA.	**INT**rons **INT**errupt (or **INT**ervene). **IN**trons stay **IN** the nucleus whereas **EX**ons **EX**it and are **EX**pressed.
Types of RNA	mRNA is the largest type of RNA. rRNA is the most abundant type of RNA. tRNA is the smallest type of RNA.	Mr²
Splicing of mRNA	Introns are precisely spliced out of primary mRNA transcripts. A lariat-shaped intermediate is formed. Small nuclear ribonucleoprotein particles (snRNP) facilitate splicing by binding to primary mRNA transcripts and forming spliceosomes.	*Lariat* = lasso.
RNA processing (eukaryotes)	Occurs in nucleus. After transcription: 1. **Capping** on 5′ end (7-methyl-G) 2. **Polyadenylation** on 3′ end (≈200 A's) 3. **Splicing** out of introns occurs Capped and tailed transcript is called **heterogeneous nuclear RNA (hnRNA)**.	Only processed RNA is transported out of the nucleus. The cap goes on a head (the beginning of the strand) and the polyA tail goes at the end of the strand. The length of the polyA tail may be proportional to the life span of the protein.
tRNA structure	75–90 nucleotides, cloverleaf form, anticodon end is opposite 3′ aminoacyl end. All tRNAs, both eukaryotic and prokaryotic, have CCA at 3′ end along with a high percentage of chemically modified bases. The amino acid is covalently bound to the 3′ end of the tRNA.	
tRNA charging	Aminoacyl-tRNA synthetase (one per aa, uses ATP) scrutinizes aa before and after it binds to tRNA. If incorrect, bond is hydrolyzed by synthetase. The aa-tRNA bond has energy for formation of peptide bond. A mischarged tRNA reads usual codon but inserts wrong amino acid.	Aminoacyl-tRNA synthetase and binding of charged tRNA to the codon are responsible for accuracy of amino acid selection.
tRNA wobble	Third nucleotide of mRNA codon "wobble" pairs, allowing formation of non–Watson-Crick base pairs. A tRNA normally reads one to three specific codons— but each codon it reads designates the same one amino acid. Economizes number of tRNAs needed.	"G-U" is wobble (gee, you wobble), rest is standard A-U and G-C. Inosine has three-way wobble: I-U, I-C, or I-A.

DNA repair defects	Xeroderma pigmentosum (skin sensitivity to UV light), ataxia-telangiectasia (x-rays), Fanconi's anemia (cross-linking agents). Repair defects are presumed.

Xeroderma pigmentosum	Defective excision repair such as uvr ABC exonuclease. Results in inability to repair thymidine dimers, which form in DNA when exposed to UV light. Associated with dry skin, melanoma and other cancers.	
Fructose intolerance	Hereditary deficiency of aldolase B. Fructose-1-phosphate accumulates, causing a decrease in available phosphate, which results in inhibition of glycogenolysis and gluconeogenesis, thus causing severe hypoglycemia.	Must decrease intake of both fructose and sucrose (glucose + fructose).
Galactosemia	Absence of galactose 1-phosphate uridyl transferase. Autosomal recessive. Damage is caused by accumulation of toxic substances (including galactitol) rather than absence of an essential compound. Symptoms: cataracts, hepatosplenomegaly, mental retardation. Treatment: exclude galactose and lactose (glactose + glucose) from diet.	
Lactase deficiency	Age-dependent and/or hereditary lactose intolerance (blacks, Asians). Symptoms: bloating, cramps, osmotic diarrhea. Treatment: avoid milk or add lactase pills to diet.	
Pyruvate dehydrogenase deficiency	Causes backup of substrate (pyruvate and alanine), resulting in lactic acidosis. Findings: neurologic defects. Treatment: increased intake of ketogenic nutrients.	Lysine and leucine—the only purely ketogenic amino acids.
Glucose-6-phosphate dehydrogenase deficiency	G6PD is rate-limiting enzyme in HMP shunt (which yields NADPH). ↓ NADPH in RBCs leads to **hemolytic anemia** due to poor RBC defense against oxidizing agents (fava beans, aspirin, sulfonamides, antimalarial drugs) and anti-tuberculosis drugs. X-linked recessive disorder.	G6PD deficiency more prevalent among blacks. NADPH is necessary to keep glutathione reduced, which in turn keeps the heme iron reduced so that O_2 can bind.
Glycolytic enzyme deficiency	Hexokinase, glucose-phosphate isomerase, aldolase, triose-phosphate isomerase, phosphate-glycerate kinase, and enolase deficiencies are associated with hemolytic anemia.	RBCs depend on glycolysis (energy and reducing equivalents).

Glycogen storage diseases

12 types, all resulting in abnormal glycogen metabolism and an accumulation of glycogen within cells.

Von Gierke's: liver.
McArdle's: muscle.
Pompe's: liver, heart, and muscle.

Type I

Von Gierke's disease = glucose 6-phosphatase deficiency. Findings: severe fasting hypoglycemia, ↑↑ glycogen in liver.

Type II

Pompe's disease = lysosomal α-1,4, glucosidase deficiency.
Findings: cardiomegaly and systemic findings, leading to early death.

Type V

McArdle's disease = muscle glycogen phosphorylase deficiency.
Findings: ↑ glycogen in muscle, but cannot break it down, leading to painful cramps, myoglobinuria with strenuous exercise.

Hartnup's disease

Defect in GI uptake of neutral amino acids. Symptoms mimic pellagra (diarrhea, dementia, dermatitis) because of malabsorption of tryptophan (precursor of niacin). Carcinoid syndrome may also cause pellagra.

Hard-N-Up = Hard Neutral Uptake

Homocystinuria

Defect in cystathionine synthase. Two forms:
1. Deficiency (treatment: ↓ Met and ↑ Cys in diet)
2. Decreased affinity of synthase for pyridoxal phosphate (treatment: ↑↑ vitamin B_6 in diet)

Results in excess homocystine in the urine. Cystine becomes essential.

Maple syrup urine

Blocked degradation of **branched** amino acids (Leu, Ile, Val).
LIV
Causes severe CNS defects, mental retardation, and death.

Urine smells like maple syrup. Think of cutting (blocking) **branches** of a maple tree.

Phenylketonuria

Normally, phenylalanine is converted into tyrosine (nonessential aa). In PKU, there is ↓ phenylalanine hydroxylase or ↓ tetrahydrobiopterin cofactor. Tyrosine becomes essential and phenylalanine builds up, leading to excess phenylketones.
Findings: mental retardation, fair skin, eczema, musty body odor.
Treatment: ↓ phenylalanine and ↑ tyrosine in diet (no Nutrasweet).

Screened for at birth. Phenylketones = phenylacetate, phenyllactate, and phenylpyruvate in urine.

Alkaptonuria

Congenital deficiency of homogentisic acid oxidase in the degradative pathway of tyrosine. Resulting alkapton bodies cause dark urine. Also, the connective tissue is dark. Benign disease.

Alkapton = alkali-hapten bodies (homogentisic acid) bind to alkali. These are in the urine.

Albinism	Congenital deficiency of tyrosinase. Results in an inability to synthesize melanin from tyrosine. Can result from a lack of migration of neural crest cells.	Lack of melanin results in an increased risk of skin cancer.
Adenosine deaminase deficiency	ADA deficiency can cause **SCID**. Excess ATP and dATP imbalances nucleotide pool via feedback inhibition of ribonucleotide reductase. This prevents DNA synthesis and thus lowers lymphocyte count. First disease to be treated by experimental human gene therapy.	**SCID** = **S**evere **C**ombined (T and B) **I**mmunodeficiency **D**isease. SCID happens to kids.
Lesch-Nyhan syndrome	Purine salvage problem owing to absence of HGPRTase, which converts hypoxanthine to inosine monophosphate (IMP) and guanine to guanosine monophosphate (GMP). X-linked recessive. Findings: retardation, self-mutilation, aggression, hyperuricemia, choreoathetosis.	**LNS** = **L**acks **N**ucleotide **S**alvage (purine).
Ehlers-Danlos syndrome	10 types, all resulting in faulty collagen synthesis. Skin is stretchy (hyperextensible) with poor wound healing, joints are hypermobile. Inheritance varies from autosomal dominant (type IV) to autosomal recessive (type VI) to X-linked recessive (type IX). Type I findings: Diaphragmatic hernia. Type IV findings: Ecchymoses, arterial rupture. Type VI findings: Retinal detachment, corneal rupture.	Sounds like "feller's damn loose" (loose joints).

Sphingolipidoses

Fabry's disease	Caused by deficiency of α-galactosidase A, resulting in accumulation of ceramide trihexoside. Finding: renal failure.	X-linked recessive.
Gaucher's disease	Caused by deficiency of β-glucocerebrosidase, leading to glucocerebroside accumulation in brain, liver, spleen, and bone marrow (Gaucher's cells with characteristic "crinkled paper" enlarged cytoplasm). Type I, the more common form, is compatible with a normal life span.	Autosomal recessive.
Niemann-Pick disease	Deficiency of sphingomyelinase causes buildup of sphingomyelin and cholesterol in reticuloendothelial and parenchymal cells and tissues. Patients die by age 3.	Autosomal recessive.
Tay-Sachs disease	Absence of hexosaminidase A results in GM_2-ganglioside accumulation. Death occurs by age 3. Cherry-red spot visible on macula. Carrier rate is 1 in 30 in Jews of European descent (1 in 300 for others).	Autosomal recessive. **Tay-saX** sounds like he**X**osaminidase.

ATP Base (adenine), ribose, 3 phosphoryls. 2 phosphoanhydride bonds, 7 kcal/mol each.
Aerobic metabolism produces 38 ATP via malate shuttle, 36 ATP via G3P shuttle.
Anaerobic glycolysis produces only 2 ATP per glucose molecule.
ATP hydrolysis can be coupled to energetically unfavorable reactions.

Activated carriers Phosphoryl (ATP)
Electrons (NADH, NADPH, $FADH_2$)
Acyl (coenzyme A, lipoamide)
CO_2 (biotin)
One-carbon units (tetrahydrofolates)
CH_3 groups (SAM)
Aldehydes (TPP)
Glucose (UDP-glucose)
Choline (CDP-choline)

Extracellular messengers

Examples	Mechanism
Nicotinic receptor, norepinephrine receptor on K^+ channel in the heart	Open or close ion channels in cell membrane
Thyroid hormones, retinoic acid, steroid hormones, vitamin D_3	Act via cytoplasmic or nuclear receptors to increase transcription of target genes
Angiotensin II, α_1-receptor, ADH	Activate phospholipase C with intracellular production of DAG, IP_3, protein kinase C and Ca^{++}
β_1-receptor, β_2-receptor ($\uparrow$ cAMP), α_2-receptor ($\downarrow$ cAMP)	Activate or inhibit adenylate cyclase
ANP, nitric oxide (EDRF)	Increase cyclic GMP in the cell
Insulin, EGF, PDGF, M-CSF	Increased tyrosine kinase activity
TGF-β	Increased serine kinase activity

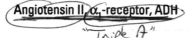

"Triple A"

NAD$^+$/NADPH **NAD$^+$** is generally used in **catabolic** processes to carry reducing equivalents away as NADH. **NADPH** is used in **anabolic** processes as a supply of reducing equivalents. NADPH is a product of the HMP shunt and the malate dehydrogenase reaction.

S-adenosyl-methionine ATP + methionine → SAM. SAM transfers methyl units to a wide variety of acceptors (e.g., in synthesis of phosphocreatine, high-energy phosphate active in muscle ATP production). Regeneration of methionine (and thus SAM) is dependent on vitamin B_{12}. SAM the methyl donor man.

Biochemistry

HIGH-YIELD FACTS

Metabolism sites

Mitochondria	Fatty acid **O**xidation, **A**cetyl-CoA production, **K**reb's cycle.	Mity **OAK**
Cytoplasm	Glycolysis, fatty acid synthesis, HMP shunt, protein synthesis (RER), steroid synthesis (SER).	
Both	Gluconeogenesis, urea cycle.	

Fructose metabolism

Fructose → fructose-1-phosphate → three-carbon intermediates, which then enter glycolysis.

Hexokinase versus glucokinase

Hexokinase is found throughout body. **Glucokinase** (lower affinity [$\uparrow K_m$] but higher capacity [$\uparrow V_{max}$]) is found only in the liver.

Hexokinase is found all over **heck**; it is feedback inhibited by G6P (glucokinase—not feedback inhibited by G6P).

Glycolysis regulation

D-glucose $\xrightarrow{\text{Hexokinase}}$ glucose 6-phosphate

Glucose 6-P $\ominus$

Fructose 6-P $\xrightarrow[\text{(rate-limiting step)}]{\text{Phosphofructokinase}}$ fructose 1,6-BP

ATP $\ominus$, AMP $\oplus$, citrate $\ominus$, fructose 2, 6-BP $\oplus$

Phosphoenolpyruvate $\xrightarrow{\text{Pyruvate kinase}}$ pyruvate

ATP $\ominus$, alanine $\ominus$, fructose 1,6-BP $\oplus$

Pyruvate $\xrightarrow{\text{Pyruvate dehydrogenase}}$ acetyl CoA

ATP $\ominus$, NADH $\ominus$, acetyl-CoA $\ominus$

Gluconeogenesis, irreversible enzymes

Pyruvate carboxylase	In mitochondria. Pyruvate → oxaloacetate.	Requires biotin, ATP. Activated by acetyl CoA. "BA"
PEP carboxykinase	In cytosol. Oxaloacetate → phosphoenolpyruvate.	Requires GTP. G"
Fructose 1,6-bisphosphatase	In cytosol. Fructose 1,6-bisphosphate → fructose 6-P	
Glucose 6-phosphatase	In cytosol. Glucose 6-P → glucose	

Above enzymes found only in liver, kidney, intestinal epithelium.

Hypoglycemia is caused by a deficiency of these key gluconeogenic enzymes listed above, e.g., von Gierke's disease, which is caused by a lack of glucose-6-phosphatase in the liver.

Pentose phosphate pathway

- Produces ribose 5-P from G6P for nucleotide synthesis.
- Produces NADPH from $NADP^+$ for fatty acid and steroid biosynthesis and for maintaining reduced glutathione inside RBCs.
  Part of HMP shunt.
  All reactions of this pathway occur in the cytoplasm.
  Sites: lactating mammary glands, liver, adrenal cortex—all sites of fatty acid or steroid synthesis.

Biochemistry

HIGH-YIELD FACTS

Cori cycle

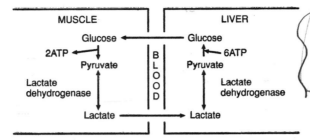

Transfers excess reducing equivalents from RBCs and muscle to liver, allowing muscle to function anaerobically (net 2 ATP).

Pyruvate dehydrogenase complex

The complex contains three enzymes that require five cofactors: NAD (niacin), FAD (riboflavin), thiamine pyrophosphate (from thiamine), lipoic acid, CoA (from pantothenate). Reaction: pyruvate + NAD^+ + CoA → acetyl CoA + CO_2 + NADH. "NFL CT"

Complex is similar to the α-ketoglutarate dehydrogenase complex (same cofactors, similar substrate and action).

TCA cycle

Pyruvate

Pyruvate dehydrog

⊖ ATP
⊖ Acetyl CoA
⊖ NADH

Acetyl-CoA

⊖ ATP

Oxalo-acetate

Citrate Synthase

Citrate

NADH

Malate

cis-Aconitate

Fumarate

Isocitrate

Isocitrate dehydrog

CO_2 + NADH

FADH$_2$

⊖ ATP
⊖ NADH
⊕ ADP

α-ketoglutarate

CO_2 + NADH

Succinate

α-KG dehydrog

GTP + CoA

Succinyl CoA

⊖ Succinyl CoA
⊖ NADH
⊖ ATP

Produces 3NADH, 1FADH$_2$, 2CO_2, 1GTP per acetyl CoA = 12ATP/acetyl CoA (2x everything per glucose)

α-Ketoglutarate dehydrogenase complex co-factors:
1. Thiamine pyrophosphate
2. Lipoamide
3. CoA
4. FAD
5. NAD^+

NFLCT

Electron transport chain and oxidative phosphorylation

NADH → NADH dehydrogenase → Q → Cytochrome bc$_1$ → Cytochrome c → Cytochrome oxidase aa$_3$ → O_2 → reduced → H_2O

Amytal Rotenone

Antimycin A

CN^-, N_3^-, CO

Oligomycin

Proton gradient → ATP

ADP+P$_i$ → Mitochondrial ATPase

FADH$_2$

Electron transport chain: 1 NADH → 3ATP; 1 FADH$_2$ → 2ATP

Oxidative phosphorylation poisons
1. Electron transport inhibitors (rotenone, antimycin A, CN^-, CO) directly inhibit electron transport causing ↓ of proton gradient and block of ATP synthesis.
2. ATPase inhibitor (oligomycin) directly inhibits mitochondrial ATPase, causing ↑ of proton gradient, but no ATP is produced because electron transport stops.
3. Uncoupling agents (2,4-DNP) increase permeability of membrane, causing ↓ of proton gradient and ↑ oxygen consumption. ATP synthesis stops. Electron transport continues.

RBC energetics	RBCs have no mitochondria (no TCA) and thus depend on glycolysis (ATP) for energy and HMP shunt (NADPH) for reducing equivalents.	Brain and RBCs rely on glucose for energy. (Brain can use ketone bodies in starvation.)
Fatty acid metabolism sites	Fatty acid synthesis = cytosol. Fatty acid degradation = mitochondria. Fatty acid entry into mitochondrion is via carnitine shuttle (inhibited by cytoplasmic malonyl-CoA).	Fatty acid degradation occurs where its products will be consumed—in the mitochondrion.
Sphingolipid components	Sphingosine precursors are serine + palmitate. Ceramide=sphingosine + fatty acid. Sphingomyelin=ceramide + phosphoryl choline. Cerebroside=ceramide + glucose/galactose. Ganglioside=ceramide + oligosaccharide + sialic acid.	
Cholesterol synthesis	Rate-limiting step is catalyzed by **HMG-CoA reductase,** which converts HMG-CoA to mevalonate. Two-thirds of plasma cholesterol is esterified by lecithin-cholesterol acyltransferase (LCAT), also known as phosphatidyl-choline: cholesterol acyltransferase (PCAT).	Lovastatin inhibits HMG-CoA reductase.

Lipoproteins

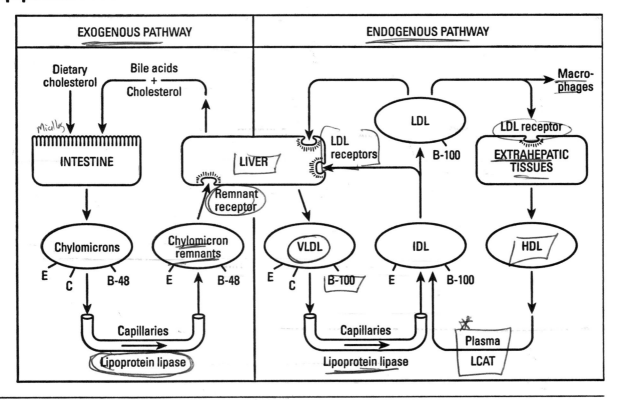

Lipoprotein functions

	Function and Route	Apolipoproteins
Chylomicrons	Deliver dietary triglycerides to peripheral tissues and dietary cholesterol to liver. Secreted by intestinal epithelial cells.	B-48 mediates secretion. A is required for formation of new HDL. C activates lipoprotein lipase. E mediates uptake of remnant by liver.
VLDL	Deliver hepatic triglycerides to peripheral tissues. Secreted by liver.	B-100 mediates secretion. C activates lipoprotein lipase. E mediates metabolism of remnant.
LDL	Deliver hepatic cholesterol to peripheral tissues. Formed by lipoprotein lipase modification of VLDL in the peripheral tissue. Taken up by target cells via receptor-mediated endocytosis.	B-100 mediates binding to cell surface receptor for endocytosis.
HDL	Mediate centripetal transport of cholesterol. Some derived from the surface components of chylomicrons. Others secreted by the liver.	LCAT catalyzes esterification of cholesterol. A activates LCAT. D mediates transfer of cholesteryl esters to other lipoprotein particles.

Aminolevulinate (ALA) synthase

Rate-limiting step for heme synthesis. The end product (heme) feedback inhibits this enzyme. Found in the mitochondria, where it converts succinyl CoA and glycine to ALA.

Heme synthesis

Occurs in the liver and bone marrow. Committed step is glycine + succinyl CoA → δ-aminolevulinate. Accumulation of intermediates causes porphyrias. Lead inhibits ALA dehydratase and ferrochelatase, causing anemia and porphyria.

Underproduced heme causes microcytic hypochromic anemia.

Heme catabolism

Heme is scavenged from RBCs and Fe^{2+} is reused. Heme → biliverdin → bilirubin (sparingly water soluble, toxic to CNS, transported by albumin). Bilirubin removed from blood by liver, conjugated with glucuronate and excreted in bile. In the intestine it is processed into its excreted form. Some urobilinogen, an intestinal intermediate, is reabsorbed into blood and excreted as urobilin into urine.

Hyperbilirubinemia	From conjugated (direct) and/or unconjugated (indirect) bilirubin. Causes: massive hemolysis, block in subsequent catabolism of heme, displacement from binding sites on albumin, e.g., liver damage or bile duct obstruction Bilirubin is yellow, causing jaundice.	**UN**conjugated is **IN**direct and **IN**soluble. Conjugated bilirubin is excreted in the urine.
Essential amino acids	Ketogenic: Leu, Lys. Glucogenic/ketogenic: Ile, Phe, Trp. Glucogenic: Met, Thr, Val, Arg, His.	**PriVaTe TIM HALL** Arg and His are required during periods of growth.
Acidic and basic amino acids	At body pH (7.4) acidic amino acids Asp and Glu are negatively charged; basic amino acids Arg and Lys are positively charged. Basic amino acid His at pH 7.4 has no net charge. Arginine is the most basic amino acid. Arg and Lys are found in high amounts in histones, which bind to negatively charged DNA.	Asp = aspartic ACID, Glu = glutamic ACID. Arg and Lys have an extra NH_3 group. The **ASP**iring **GLU**tton was **ACID**ic so others **BASIC**ally **ARG**ued with, **LY**ed to, and **HIS**sed at him.
Protein synthesis: ATP versus GTP	P site = peptidyl, A site = aminoacyl. ATP is used in tRNA charging, whereas GTP is used in binding of tRNA to ribosome and for translocation.	P = peptidyl, A = amino acid or acceptor site (on deck). Erythromycin inhibits the translocation step of protein synthesis.
Protein synthesis direction	Synthesis proceeds from N terminus to C terminus. mRNA is read $5' \rightarrow 3'$. Signal sequences are found on the N terminus of newly synthesized secretory and nuclear proteins.	The ami**N**o a**C**ids are tied together from **N** to **C**.
Urea cycle	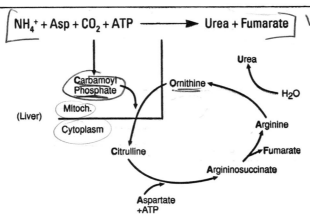	**O**rdinarily, **C**areless **C**rappers **A**re **A**lso **F**rivolous **A**bout **U**rination.

$$NH_4^+ + Asp + CO_2 + ATP \longrightarrow Urea + Fumarate$$

Biochemistry

HIGH-YIELD FACTS

Arachidonic acid products

Phospholipase A_2 liberates arachidonic acid from cell membrane. Lipoxygenase pathway yields leukotrienes. Cyclooxygenase pathway yields thromboxanes, prostaglandins, and prostacyclin. **L** for **L**ipoxygenase and **L**eukotriene.

Tx A_2 stimulates platelet aggregation.
PG I_2 inhibits platelet aggregation.
LT B_4 is a neutrophil chemoattractant.
LT C_4, D_4, and E_4 (SRS-A) function in bronchoconstriction, vasoconstriction, contraction of smooth muscle, and increased vascular permeability

Insulin

Made in β cells of pancreas. No effect on glucose uptake by brain, RBCs, and hepatocytes. Required for adipose and skeletal muscle uptake of glucose. Inhibits glucagon release by α cells of pancreas.

Brain, liver, and RBCs take up glucose independent of insulin. Insulin moves glucose into cells.

Ketone bodies

In liver: fatty acid and amino acids $\rightarrow$ acetoacetate + β-hydroxybutyrate (to be used in muscle and brain). Ketone bodies found in prolonged starvation and diabetic ketoacidosis. Excreted in urine. Made from HMG-CoA. Ketone bodies are metabolized by the brain to 2 molecules of acetyl CoA.

Breath smells like acetone (fruity odor). Urine test for ketones does not detect β-hydroxybutyrate (favored by high redox state).

Ethanol hypoglycemia

Ethanol metabolism increases NADH/NAD$^+$ ratio in liver, causing diversion of pyruvate to lactate and OAA to malate, thereby inhibiting gluconeogenesis and leading to hypoglycemia.

Ethanol metabolism

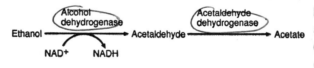

NAD$^+$ is the limiting reagent.
Alcohol dehydrogenase operates via zero order kinetics.

Disulfiram (Antabuse) inhibits acetaldehyde dehydrogenase (acetaldehyde accumulates, contributing to hangover symptoms).

Kwashiorkor versus marasmus

Kwashiorkor = protein malnutrition resulting in skin lesions, edema, liver malfunction (fatty change). Clinical picture is small child with swollen belly.
Marasmus = protein-calorie malnutrition resulting in tissue wasting.

Signal molecule precursors	ATP → cAMP via adenylate cyclase.
	GTP → cGMP via guanylate cyclase.
	Glutamate → GABA via glutamate decarboxylase (requires vit. B_6).
	Tyrosine → DOPA via tyrosine hydroxylase, the rate-limiting enzyme of catecholamine biosynthesis.
	Choline → ACh via choline acetyltransferase (ChAT).
	Arachidonate → prostaglandins, thromboxanes, leukotrienes via cyclooxygenase/lipoxygenase.
	Fructose-6-P → fructose-1,6-bis-P via phosphofructokinase (PFK), the rate-limiting enzyme of glycolysis.
	1,3-BPG → 2,3-BPG via bisphosphoglycerate mutase.

Tyrosine derivatives	Tyrosine derivatives are thyroxine, dopamine, epinephrine, melanin.	Tire-sine ("tired without") substances that get you going: thyroxine, epinephrine, dopamine (as in Parkinson's), melanin (gets you outdoors).

Enzyme kinetics

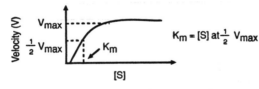

$K_m = [S]$ at $\frac{1}{2} V_{max}$

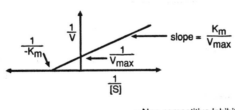

slope $= \dfrac{K_m}{V_{max}}$

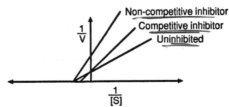

Competitive inhibitors: Resemble substrates; bind reversibly to active sites of enzymes. High substrate concentration overcomes effect of inhibitor. V_{max} remains unchanged, K_m increases compared to uninhibited.

Noncompetitive inhibitors: Do not resemble substrate; bind to enzyme but not at active site. Inhibition cannot be overcome by high substrate concentration. V_{max} decreases, K_m remains unchanged compared to uninhibited.

HIGH-YIELD FACTS

Biochemistry

Cell cycle phases

M (mitosis: prophase–metaphase–anaphase–telophase)
G_1 (growth)
S (synthesis of DNA)
G_2 (growth)
G_0 (quiescent G_1 phase)
G_1 and G_0 are of variable duration. Mitosis is usually shortest phase. Most cells are in G_0.

G stands for **gap** or **growth**, **S** for synthesis.

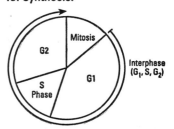

Plasma membrane composition

Plasma membranes contain cholesterol (≈50%, promotes membrane stability), phospholipids (≈50%), sphingolipids, glycolipids, and proteins. Only noncytoplasmic side of membrane contains glycosylated lipids or proteins (i.e., the plasma membrane is an asymmetric, fluid bilayer).

Phosphatidylcholine function

Phosphatidylcholine (lecithin) is a major component of RBC membranes, of myelin, of bile, and of surfactant (DPPC–dipalmitoylphosphatidylcholine).

Keratin composition and function

Keratin is a protein with a high percentage of cysteine. It is found in intermediate filaments (nails and keratinized squamous epithelium).

Microtubule

Cylindrical structure 23 nm in diameter and of variable length. A helical array of polymerized dimers of α- and β-tubulin (13 per circumference). Each dimer has 2 GTP bound. Incorporated into flagella, cilia, mitotic spindles. Grows slowly, collapses quickly. Microtubules are also involved in slow axoplasmic transport in neurons.

Drugs that act on microtubules include colchicine (anti-gout), vinblastine/vincristine and taxol (anti-cancer), griseofulvin (anti-fungal), and mebendazole/thiabendazole (anti-helminthic). Colchicine inhibits microtubule polymerization. Vincristine and vinblastine interact with tubulin to block assembly of mitotic spindle.

Collagen structure

Collagen fibril = many staggered collagen molecules (linked by lysyl oxidase). Collagen molecule = 3 collagen α chains (usually X-Y-Gly, X and Y = proline, hydroxyproline, or hydroxylysine). Procollagen must be trimmed to collagen molecule.

Cholesterol lipoproteins

LDL and HDL carry most cholesterol. LDL transports cholesterol from liver to tissue; HDL tranports it from periphery to liver.

HDL is Healthy.
LDL is Lousy.

Biochemistry

HIGH-YIELD FACTS

Hemoglobin	Hemoglobin is composed of four polypeptide subunits (2α and 2β) and exists in two forms: 1. T (taut) form has low affinity for oxygen. 2. R (relaxed) form has high affinity for oxygen ($300\times$). Hemoglobin exhibits positive cooperativity and negative allostery (accounts for the sigmoid-shaped O_2 dissociation curve for hemoglobin), unlike myoglobin.	Carbon monoxide has a $200\times$ greater affinity for hemoglobin than oxygen.
Hb structure regulation	Increased Cl^-, H^+, CO_2, DPG and temperature favor T form over R form (shifts dissociation curve to right, leading to $\uparrow O_2$ unloading). T form has low affinity for O_2.	When you're Relaxed, you do your job better (carry O_2).
CO_2 transport in blood	CO_2 binds to amino acids in globin chain (at N terminus) but not to heme. CO_2 binding favors T (taut) form of hemoglobin (and thus promotes O_2 unloading).	CO_2 must be transported from tissue to lungs, the reverse of O_2.
Hormonal effects on cAMP	Insulin reduces cAMP levels. Epinephrine, norepinephrine, and glucagon raise cAMP levels.	cAMP mobilizes resources (remember ATP → cAMP).
PIP_2 second messenger system	Involved in mast cell degranulation, α_1 receptor activation, and activation of some muscarinic receptors.	PIP_2 $\nearrow$ IP_3 → $\uparrow Ca^{2+}$ (from ER) $\searrow$ DAG → protein kinase
Muscle activation: calcium	In skeletal muscle, calcium ions activate troponin, which moves tropomyosin, which exposes and activates actin. In smooth muscle, Ca^{2+} activates contraction by binding to calmodulin (no troponins).	
Sodium pump	Na^+-K^+ATPase is located in the plasma membrane with ATP site on cytoplasmic side. For each ATP consumed, 3 Na^+ go out and 2 K^+ come in. During cycle, pump is phosphorylated (vanadate inhibited). Ouabain inhibits by binding to K^+ site. Cardiac glycosides (digoxin, digitoxin) also inhibit the Na^+-K^+ATPase, causing increased cardiac contractility.	
Enzyme regulation methods	Enzyme concentration alteration (synthesis and/or destruction), covalent modification (e.g., phosphorylation), proteolytic modification (zymogen), allosteric regulation (e.g., feedback inhibition), and transcriptional regulation (e.g., steroid hormones).	

BIOCHEMISTRY—VITAMINS

Vitamin A (retinol)

Deficiency	Night blindness and dry skin.	Retinol is vitamin A, so think
Function	Constituent of visual pigments (retinal).	Retin-A (used topically for
Excess	Arthralgias, fatigue, headaches, skin changes.	wrinkles and acne).

Biochemistry

HIGH-YIELD FACTS

Vitamin B₁ (thiamine)

the "T" of NFL CT

Deficiency	Beriberi and Wernicke-Korsakoff syndrome.
Function	In thiamine pyrophosphate, a cofactor for oxidative decarboxylation of α-keto acids (pyruvate, α-ketoglutarate) and a cofactor for transketolase.

Beriberi: characterized by polyneuritis, cardiac pathology, and edema. Spell beriberi as **Ber1Ber1**.
Wet beriberi may lead to high output cardiac failure.

Vitamin B₂ (riboflavin)

Deficiency	Angular stomatitis.
Function	Cofactor in oxidation and reduction (e.g., $FADH_2$).

FAD and FMN are derived from riboFlavin.
NAD derived from Niacin.

Niacin (B₃)

Deficiency	Pellagra.
Function	Constituent of NAD^+, $NADP^+$ (used in redox reactions). Derived from tryptophan.

Pellagra's symptoms are the **3 Ds**: Diarrhea, Dermatitis, Dementia (also beefy glossitis).

Vitamin B₅ (pantothenate)

Deficiency	Dermatitis, enteritis, alopecia, adrenal insufficiency.
Function	Constituent of CoA, part of fatty acid synthase. Cofactor for acyl transfers.

Pantothen-A is in Co-A.

Vitamin B₆ (pyridoxine)

Deficiency	Convulsions, hyperirritability (inducible by INH).
Function	Converted to pyridoxal phosphate, a cofactor used in transamination (e.g., ALT and AST), decarboxylation, and transsulfuration.

Biotin

Deficiency	Dermatitis, enteritis.
Function	Cofactor for carboxylations but not decarboxylations.

Buy-a-tin of CO_2 for carboxylations.

Folic acid

Deficiency	Macrocytic, megaloblastic anemia (often no neurologic symptoms), sprue.
Function	Coenzyme for one-carbon transfer; involved in methylation reactions. Important for the synthesis of nitrogenous bases in DNA and RNA.

Eat green leaves (since folic acid is not stored very long).
PABA is the folic acid precursor in bacteria. Sulfa drugs and dapsone are PABA analogs.

Vitamin B₁₂ (cobalamin)

Deficiency   Macrocytic, megaloblastic anemia, neurologic symptoms.

Function
- Cofactor for homocysteine methylation and methyl-malonyl-CoA handling.
- Stored primarily in the liver.
- Synthesized only by microorganisms.

Vit. B₁₂ deficiency is usually caused by malabsorption (sprue, enteritis, *Diphyllobothrium latum*) or no intrinsic factor (pernicious anemia).

Vitamin C (ascorbic acid)

Deficiency   Scurvy.

Function
- Necessary for hydroxylation of proline and lysine in collagen synthesis.
- Scurvy findings: swollen gums, bruising, anemia, poor wound healing.

Vitamin **C** Cross-links **C**ollagen. British sailors carried limes to prevent scurvy.

Vitamin D

D₂ = ergocalciferol, consumed in milk.
D₃ = cholecalciferol, formed in sun-exposed skin.

Deficiency   Rickets in children (bending bones), osteomalacia in adults (soft bones), and hypocalcemic tetany.

Function   Increases intestinal absorption of calcium and phosphate.

Excess   Hypercalcemia, loss of appetite, stupor. Seen in sarcoidosis, a disease where the epithelioid macrophages convert vit. D into its active form.

Remember that drinking milk (fortified with vitamin D) is good for bones.

Vitamin E

Deficiency   Increased fragility of erythrocytes.

Function   Antioxidant (protects erythrocytes from hemolysis).

Vitamin K

Deficiency   Neonatal hemorrhage with ↑ PT, ↑ PTT, but normal bleeding time.

Function   Catalyzes γ-carboxylation of glutamic acid residues on various proteins concerned with blood clotting. Synthesized by intestinal flora. Therefore, vit. K deficiency can occur after the prolonged use of broad-spectrum antibiotics.

K for **K**oagulation. Note that the vitamin K-dependent clotting factors are II, VII, IX, and X. Warfarin is a vitamin K antagonist.

Vitamins: fat soluble

A, D, E, K. Absorption dependent on gut (ileum) and pancreas. Toxicity more common than for water-soluble vitamins, since these accumulate in fat.

Malabsorption of fat-soluble vitamins, which can be caused by conditions such as cystic fibrosis, results in sprue. Mineral oil (laxative) can also cause malabsorption of fat-soluble vitamins.

HIGH-YIELD FACTS

Biochemistry

Vitamins: water soluble

B_1 (thiamine: TPP)
B_2 (riboflavin: FAD, FMN)
B_5 (pantothenate: CoA)
B_6 (pyridoxine: PP)
B_{12} (cobalamin)
Niacin (nicotinate: NAD^+)
C (ascorbic acid)
Biotin
Folate

All wash out easily from body except B_{12} (stored in liver).

DNA/RNA/Protein

1. Common tools of molecular biology (e.g., restriction enzymes, cloning vectors, and cDNA libraries) and their applications.
2. Basic principles and interpretation of new molecular biology techniques (e.g., PCR, restriction fragment polymorphism, Southern blotting, Northern blotting, and Western blotting).
3. The operon model of DNA regulation.
4. Events of protein synthesis, processing, and secretion.
5. Acid-base titration curve (pK_a, pI).

Genetic Errors

1. Diseases caused by mineral deficiencies (e.g., iron, magnesium).
2. Classification and treatment of the major types of inherited hyperlipidemia.
3. Hemoglobinopathies (e.g., thalassemias, sickle cell anemia).

Metabolism

1. Regulation of glycogen synthesis.
2. Oxygen consumption, carbon dioxide production, and ATP production for fats, proteins, and carbohydrates.
3. Amino acid degradation pathways (urea cycle and tricarboxylic acid cycle).
4. Phosphorylative steps in metabolic pathways.
5. Regulation of rate-limiting enzymes of metabolic pathways (e.g., pyruvate carboxylase).
6. Organ and cellular sites of metabolic pathways.
7. Pathways of heme synthesis and breakdown.
8. The biochemistry of fat absorption and metabolism.
9. Forms of energy utilized by the brain, muscle, and other organs in postprandial versus fasting subjects.
10. Important tyrosine kinases, including growth factor receptors (e.g., insulin and EGF receptors).
11. Synthesis and metabolism of neurotransmitters (e.g., acetylcholine, epinephrine, norepinephrine, dopamine).
12. Effects of insulin on cellular and tissue metabolism.

Microbiology

This high-yield material covers the basic concepts of microbiology and immunology. The emphasis in previous examinations has been approximately 40% bacteriology (20% basic, 20% quasi-clinical), 25% immunology, 25% virology (10% basic, 15% quasi-clinical), 5% parasitology, and 5% mycology. Memorizing the distinguishing characteristics, target organs, and method of spread of, as well as relevant laboratory tests for, major pathogens can improve your score substantially.

Many students preparing for this part of the boards make the mistake of studying bacteriology very well without devoting sufficient time to the other topics. For this reason, learning immunology and virology well is high yield. Learn the components of the immune response, including T cells, B cells, and the structure and functions of immunoglobulins as well as immunodeficiency diseases (eg, agammaglobulinemia, DiGeorge's syndrome). Knowledge of viral structures and genomes is also very important.

Bugs

Viruses

Immunology

High-Yield Topics

Auxotroph, autotroph, heterotroph

Auxotroph	Nutritionally deficient species. Require nutrients not required by parental or prototype strain.	**Aux.** troph requires **aux**iliary nourishment.
Heterotroph	Require carbon source, sugar, or amino acids.	All human pathogens are heterotrophs.
Autotroph	Require only CO_2 and energy source.	

Obligate aerobes

Examples include *Pseudomonas aeruginosa* and *Mycobacterium tuberculosis*.
Mycobacterium tuberculosis has a predilection for the apices of the lung, because the apices have the highest Po_2.

*P. **AER**uginosa* is an **AER**obe seen in burn wounds, nosocomial pneumonia, and pneumonias in cystic fibrosis patients.

Obligate anaerobes

Examples include *Clostridium, Bacteroides*. They lack catalase and/or superoxide dismutase and thus are susceptible to oxidative damage. They are generally foul-smelling (short-chain fatty acids), difficult to culture, and produce gas in tissue (CO_2 and H_2).

Anaerobes are normal flora in GI tract, pathogenic elsewhere. Aminoglycosides ineffective against anaerobes since these antibiotics require O_2 to enter into bacterial cell.

Bacterial growth curve

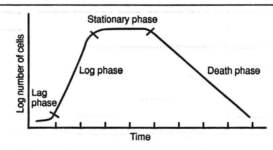

Microbiology

HIGH-YIELD FACTS

Bacterial structures

Structure	Function	Chemical composition
Peptidoglycan	Gives rigid support, protects against osmotic pressure	Sugar backbone with cross-linked peptide side chains
Outer membrane (gram positives)	Major surface antigen	Teichoic acid
Outer membrane (gram negatives)	Toxic moiety of endotoxin Major surface antigen	Lipid A Polysaccharide
Plasma membrane	Site of oxidative and transport enzymes	Lipoprotein bilayer
Ribosome	Protein synthesis	RNA and protein in 50S and 30S subunits
Nucleoid	Genetic material	DNA
Mesosome	Participates in cell division	Invagination of plasma membrane
Periplasm	Space between the cytoplasmic membrane and outer membrane	Contains many hydrolytic enzymes, including β-lactamases
Capsule	Protects against phagocytosis	Polysaccharide (except *Bacillus anthracis*)
Pilus/fimbria	Mediates adherence of bacteria to cell surface and attachment to bacteria during conjugation	Glycoprotein
Flagellum	Motility	Protein
Spore	Provides resistance to dehydration, heat, and chemicals	Keratin-like coat Dipicolinic acid
Plasmid	Contains a variety of genes for antibiotic resistance, enzymes, and toxins	DNA
Glycocalyx	Mediates adherence to surfaces, especially foreign surfaces (e.g., indwelling catheters)	Polysaccharide

Spores: bacterial	Only certain gram-positive rods form spores when nutrients are limited. Spores are highly resistant to destruction by heat and chemicals . Have dipicolinic acid in their walls. Have no metabolic activity. Must autoclave to kill spores.	Gram-positive soil bugs ≈ spore formers (*Bacillus anthracis*, *Clostridium perfringens*, *C. tetani*).
Spores: fungal	Most fungal spores are asexual. Both coccidioidomycosis and histoplasmosis are transmitted by inhalation of asexual spores. Ascospores from ascomycetes are sexual.	Conidia ≡ asexual fungal spores (e.g., blastoconidia, arthroconidia).
Antigenic variation	Classic examples: Bacteria: *Salmonella* (two flagellar variants), *Borrelia* (relapsing fever), *Neisseria gonorrhoeae* (pilus protein). Virus: influenza (major = shift, minor = drift). Parasites: trypanosomes (predictable sequence).	Some mechanisms for variation include DNA rearrangement and RNA segment rearrangement (e.g., influenza major shift).

HIGH-YIELD FACTS

Microbiology

Microbiology

HIGH-YIELD FACTS

Bacterial genetic transfer	Conjugation ≡ direct DNA transfer via sex (fertility, F) pilus.	Conjugation = with joining.
	Transduction ≡ DNA transfer via bacteriophage vector.	Transduction ≈ trans-**DUCK**-tion (imagine duck vector carrying DNA in bill).
	Transformation ≡ uptake of naked DNA from environment.	Transformation ≈ trans-**FROM**-ation (from environment).
	Transposon ≡ "jumping genes," DNA sequences that jump from bacterium to bacterium or from bacterium to plasmid.	

Exotoxins	Peptides that are excreted by both gram-positive and gram-negative bugs. They are highly antigenic and generally not associated with fever. They are relatively unstable to heat, are highly toxic, and have specific receptors. Usually encoded by lysogenic phage DNA.	**EX**otoxins are **EX**creted. Examples include tetanospasmin, botulinum toxin, and diphtheria toxin.

Bugs with exotoxins

Gram-positive bugs	**Mode of action**
Corynebacterium diphtheriae	Inactivates EF-2 by ADP ribosylation
Clostridium tetani	Blocks the release of the inhibitory neurotransmitter glycine
Clostridium botulinum	Blocks the release of acetylcholine: causes anti-cholinergic symptoms, CNS paralysis; spores found in canned food, honey (get floppy baby)
Clostridium perfringens	Alpha toxin is a lecithinase in gas gangrene. Get double zone of hemolysis on blood agar
Bacillus anthracis	One of the toxins is an adenylate cyclase
Staphylococcus aureus	Toxin is a superantigen that binds to class II MHC protein and T cell receptor, inducing IL-1 and IL-2 synthesis in toxic shock syndrome
Streptococcus pyogenes	Erythrogenic toxin (causes rash of scarlet fever) and streptolysin O (antigen for ASO-antibody present in rheumatic fever). Erythrogenic toxin is a superantigen; streptolysin O is a hemolysin
Gram-negative bugs	
Escherichia coli	Heat-labile toxin stimulates adenylate cyclase by ADP ribosylation of G protein Heat-stable toxin stimulates guanylate cyclase
Vibrio cholerae	Stimulates adenylate cyclase by ADP ribosylation of G protein; ↑ pumping of Cl⁻ and H_2O into gut.
Bordetella pertussis	Stimulates adenylate cyclase by ADP ribosylation; causes whooping cough, lymphocytosis.

Endotoxin	A lipopolysaccharide, found only in cell wall of gram-negative bacteria. Lipid A is the toxic part. Can cause hemorrhagic tissue necrosis (via TNF), DIC, fever (via IL-1), shock, metabolic acidosis; also activates complement (via alternative pathway).	e**N**dotoxin in integral part of gram-**N**egative cell wall. Endotoxin is heat stable.

108

Endotoxins vs. exotoxins

	Exotoxin	Endotoxin
Source	Some gram-positive and gram-negative bacteria	Cell wall of most gram-negative bacteria
Secreted from cell	Yes	No
Composition	Polypeptide	Lipopolysaccharide (LPS)
Location of genes	Plasmid or bacteriophage	Bacterial chromosome
Clinical effects	Various effects	Fever, shock, DIC
Mode of action	Various modes	Induces TNF and IL-1 synthesis
Vaccines	Toxoids used as vaccines (highly antigenic)	No toxoids formed and no vaccine available (poorly antigenic)

Gram stain limitations

These bugs do not gram stain well:
Treponema (too thin to be visualized)
Rickettsia (intracellular parasite)
Mycobacteria (high-lipid-content cell wall requires acid-fast stain)
Mycoplasma (no cell wall)
Legionella pneumophila (primarily intracellular)
Chlamydia (intracellular parasite)

Mycobacteria—acid fast.
Legionella—silver stain.
Treponemes—dark-field microscopy and fluorescent antibody staining.

"**T**hese **R**ascals **M**ay **M**icroscopically **L**ack **C**olor"

Fermentation patterns of *Neisseria*

The pathogenic *Neisseria* species are differentiated on the basis of sugar fermentation.

Meningococci ferment **M**altose/Glucose;
Gonococci ferment Glucose.

Pigment-producing bacteria

Staphylococcus aureus produces a yellow pigment.
Pseudomonas aeruginosa produces a blue-green pigment.
Serratia marcescens produces a red pigment.

Latin: *aureus* = gold

IgA proteases

IgA proteases allow these organisms to colonize mucosal surfaces: *Streptococcus pneumoniae*, *Neisseria meningitidis*, *Neisseria gonorrhoeae*, *Hemophilus influenzae*.

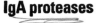 encapsulated

β-hemolytic bacteria

Include the following organisms:
1. *Staphylococcus aureus* (catalase and coagulase positive)
2. *Streptococcus pyogenes* (catalase negative and bacitracin sensitive)
3. *Streptococcus agalactiae* (catalase negative and bacitracin resistant)
4. *Listeria monocytogenes* (tumbling motility, meningitis in newborns, unpasteurized milk.)

 see Mech Infect, chart!

Microbiology

HIGH-YIELD FACTS

Catalase/coagulase (gram-positive cocci)	Catalase degrades H_2O_2, an antimicrobial product of PMNs. Staphylococci make catalase, whereas streptococci do not. *S. aureus* makes coagulase, whereas *S. epidermidis* does not.	Staph make catalase because they have more "staff." Bad staph (*aureus,* since *epidermidis* is skin flora) make coagulase and toxins.
Staphylococcus aureus	Protein A (virulence factor) binds Fc-IgG, which inhibits complement fixation and phagocytosis. *Staphylococcus aureus* produces exfoliation (scalded skin syndrome), TSST-1 (toxic shock syndrome), hemolysins, enterotoxins (food poisoning), and coagulase.	TSST is a superantigen that binds to class II MHC and T-cell receptor, resulting in polyclonal T-cell activation.
β-hemolytic strep sequelae	Pharyngeal infection can lead to acute rheumatic fever (fever, polyarthritis, carditis, elevated ASO titer). Skin infection (also known as erysipelas or impetigo) can lead to acute glomerulonephritis (elevated ASO titer, low C3).	Pharyngitis gives you rheumatic "phever."
M protein	An antiphagocytic virulence factor on cell wall of *Streptococcus pyogenes* (strep Group A). Antibody to **M** protein enhances host defenses against *S. pyogenes*.	"AM/PM"
Enterococci	Enterococci (*Streptococcus faecalis* and *S. faecium*) are penicillin G-resistant and cause UTI and subacute endocarditis. Lancefield Group D includes the enterococci and the non-enterococcal Group D streptococci. Lancefield grouping is based on differences in the C-carbohydrate on the bacterial cell wall.	*Entero* = intestine, *faecalis* = feces, *strepto* = twisted (chains), *coccus* = berry. Enterococci, hardier than nonenterococci Group D, can thus grow in 6.5% NaCl (lab test).

Diarrhea

Species	Typical findings	Fever/leukocytosis
Escherichia coli	Ferments lactose	No
Vibrio cholerae	Comma-shaped organisms	No
Salmonella	Does not ferment lactose, motile	Yes
Shigella	Does not ferment lactose, nonmotile, very low ID_{50}	Yes
Campylobacter jejuni	Comma- or S-shaped organisms; growth at 42°C	Yes
Vibrio parahaemolyticus	Transmitted by seafood	Yes
Yersinia enterocolitica	Usually transmitted from pets (e.g., puppies)	Yes

Viridans group streptococci	Viridans streptococci are α-hemolytic. They are normal flora of the oropharynx and cause dental caries (*Streptococcus mutans*) and bacterial endocarditis (*S. sanguis*). Resistant to optochin, differentiating them from *S. pneumoniae*, which is α-hemolytic but is optochin sensitive.	*Sanguis* (L) = blood. There is lots of blood in the heart (endocarditis). Viridans group strep live in the mouth because they are not afraid of-the-chin (op-to-chin resistant).

Clostridia (with exotoxins)	All gram-positive, spore-forming, anaerobic bacilli. *Clostridium tetani* produces an exotoxin causing tetanus. *C. botulinum* produces a preformed, heat-labile toxin that inhibits ACh release, causing botulism. *C. perfringens* produces α toxin, a hemolytic lecithinase that causes myonecrosis or gas gangrene. *C. difficile* produces a cytotoxin, an exotoxin that kills enterocytes, causing pseudomembranous colitis.	Tetanus is **te**tanic paralysis (blocks glycine, an inhibitory neurotransmitter). ***Botulinum*** is from bad **bott**les of food (causes a flaccid paralysis) ***perfringens* perf**orates a gangrenous leg, ***difficile*** causes **di**arrhea.
Diphtheria (and exotoxin)	Caused by *Corynebacterium diphtheriae* via exotoxin encoded by β-prophage. Potent exotoxin inhibits protein synthesis via ADP-ribosylation of EF-2. Symptoms include pseudomembranous pharyngitis (grayish-white membrane) with lymphadenopathy. Lab diagnosis based on gram-positive rods with metachromatic granules.	**ABCDEFG:** **A**denopathy **B**eta-prophage **C**orynebacterium **D**iphtheriae **E**longation Factor 2 **G**ranules *Coryne* = club shaped. Grows on tellurite agar.
Actinomycetes	Actinomycetes are bacteria (prokaryotes) that form filaments resembling hyphae of fungi (eukaryotes).	*Actino* = ray, radiating (as in the filaments they form).
Actinomyces* versus *Nocardia	*Actinomyces israelii,* a gram-positive anaerobe, causes oral/facial abscesses with "sulfur granules" that may drain through sinus tracts in skin. *Nocardia asteroides,* a gram-positive and also a weakly acid-fast aerobe in soil, causes pulmonary infection in immunocompromised patients.	*A. israelii* forms "sulfur" granules in sinus tracts. ***Nocardia*** has **no car**, so it walks fast on acid (acid fast) and on soil but gets out of breath (pulmonary infection).
Penicillin and gram-negative bugs	Gram-negative bugs are resistant to benzyl penicillin G but may be susceptible to penicillin derivatives like ampicillin. The gram-negative outer membrane layer inhibits entry of penicillin G and vancomycin.	
Periplasmic space	Space between outer membrane and cytoplasmic membrane in gram-negative bacteria. Periplasm contains enzymes (e.g., β-lactamases such as penicillinases).	Only gram-negatives have a periplasmic space.
Bugs causing food poisoning	*Vibrio parahaemolyticus* in contaminated seafood. *Bacillus cereus* in reheated rice. *Staphylococcus aureus* in meats. *Clostridium perfringens* in reheated meat dishes.	**V**omit **B**ig **S**melly **C**hunks.

Microbiology

HIGH-YIELD FACTS

Enterobacteriaceae: antigens	All species have somatic (O) antigen (which is the polysaccharide of endotoxin). The capsular (K) antigen is related to the virulence of the bug. The flagellar (H) antigen is found in motile species. All ferment glucose and are oxidase negative (except *Pseudomonas aeruginosa*, which is oxidase positive).	Think **KOH:** **K**apsular s**O**matic flag**H**ellar. (Or think flagella spin like **H**elicopter blades.)
Haemophilus influenzae	Causes meningitis, otitis media, pneumonia, epiglottitis. Small gram-negative (coccobacillary) rod. Aerosol transmission. Most invasive disease caused by capsular type b. Produces IgA protease. Culture on chocolate agar, requires factors V (NAD) and X (hemin) for growth. Treat meningitis with ceftriaxone. Rifampin prophylaxis in close contacts.	When a child has flu, mom goes to five (V) and dime (X) store to buy some chocolate. Vaccine contains type b capsular polysaccharide conjugated to diphtheria toxoid or other protein. Given between 2 and 18 months of age.
Legionella pneumophila	Legionnaire's disease ("atypical" pneumonia). Gram-negative rod. Gram stains poorly—use silver stain. Grow on charcoal yeast extract culture buffered with iron and cysteine. Aerosol transmission from environmental water source habitat. No person-to-person transmission. Treat with erythromycin.	Think of a French legionnaire (soldier) with his **silver** helmet, sitting around a campfire **(charcoal)**, with his **iron** dagger—he is no sissy **(cysteine).**
Pseudomonas aeruginosa	Causes wound and burn infections, UTI, pneumonia (especially in cystic fibrosis), sepsis (black lesions on skin), external otitis (swimmer's ear), hot tub folliculitis. Aerobic gram-negative rod. Non-lactose fermenting, oxidase positive. Produces pyocyanin (blue-green) pigment. Water source. Produces endotoxin (fever, shock) and exotoxin A (inactivates EF-2). Treat with aminoglycoside plus extended-spectrum penicillin (eg, piperacillin, ticarcillin).	**AER**uginosa—**AER**obic; Think water connection and blue-green pigment.
Helicobacter pylori	Causes gastritis. Risk factor for peptic ulcer, gastric carcinoma. Gram-negative rod. Urease positive. Creates alkaline environment. Treat with triple therapy: bismuth (Pepto-Bismol), metronidazole, and either tetracycline or amoxicillin.	Pylori—think pyloris of stomach. *Proteus* and *H. pylori* are both urease positive (cleave urea to ammonia).
Lactose-fermenting enteric bacteria	These bacteria grow pink colonies on MacConkey's agar. Examples include *Citrobacter*, *E. coli*, *Enterobacter*, and *Klebsiella*.	They **"CEEK"** (seek) lactose.

Salmonella have flagella → motile

Salmonella* versus *Shigella	Both are non–lactose fermenters; both invade intestinal mucosa and cause bloody diarrhea. Only *Salmonella* is motile and can invade further and disseminate hematogenously. Symptoms of salmonellosis may be prolonged with antibiotic treatments.	Salmon swim (motile and disseminate). *Salmonella* has an animal reservoir; *Shigella* does not and is transmitted via "food, fingers, feces, and flies."
Bugs causing watery diarrhea	Include *Vibrio cholerae* (associated with rice-water stools), enterotoxigenic *E. coli,* viruses (e.g., rotaviruses), and protozoans (e.g., *Cryptosporidium* and *Giardia*).	
Bugs causing bloody diarrhea	Include *Salmonella, Shigella, Campylobacter jejuni,* enterohemorrhagic/enteroinvasive *E. coli, Yersinia enterocolitica,* and *Entamoeba histolytica* (a protozoan).	
Cholera and pertussis toxins	*Vibrio cholerae* toxin permanently activates G_s, causing rice-water diarrhea. Pertussis toxin permanently disables G_i, causing whooping cough. Both toxins act via ADP ribosylation that permanently activates adenyl cyclase (resulting in ↑ cAMP).	Cholera turns the "on" on. Pertussis turns the "off" off. Pertussis toxin also promotes lymphocytosis.

Zoonotic bacteria

Species	Disease	Source and transmission
Francisella tularensis	Tularemia	Tick bite. Sources are rabbits and deer.
Yersinia pestis	Plague	Flea bite. Sources are rodents (especially prairie dogs).
Pasteurella multocida	Cellulitis	Bites from cats and dogs, who are also the sources.
Borrelia burgdorferi	Lyme disease	Bite of *Ixodes* ticks that live on mice and deer.

Undulant fever/ brucellosis	Caused by ingestion of unpasteurized dairy products contaminated with *Brucella abortus* (cattle) or *B. melitensis* (goats) or contact with animals (goats, cattle, pigs). *Brucella* can replicate within macrophages. Undulant fever is an occupational hazard for butchers and meat handlers. Treat with tetracycline.	Picture ungulates (hoofed mammals) "hoofing it up" in your macrophages—**un**gulates give you **un**dulant fever.

Intracellular bugs

Obligate intracellular	*Rickettsia, Chlamydia*	Stay inside (cells) when it is "**R**eally **C**old."
Facultative intracellular	*Mycobacterium, Brucella, Francisella, Listeria*	

Mycobacteria: atypical	*Mycobacterium kansasii* (pulmonary TB-like symptoms). *M. scrofulaceum* (cervical lymphadenitis in kids). *M. avium-intracellulare* (often resistant to multiple drugs; causes disseminated disease in AIDS). All mycobacteria are acid-fast organisms.

HIGH-YIELD FACTS

Microbiology

Leprosy (Hansen's disease)

Caused by *Mycobacterium leprae,* an acid-fast bacillus that likes cool temperatures (infects skin and superficial nerves), and cannot be grown in vitro. Reservoir in U.S.: armadillos.

Treatment: long-term oral dapsone; toxicity is hemolysis and metHb.

Alternate treatments include rifampin and combination of clofazimine and dapsone.

Hansen's disease has two forms: lepromatous and tuberculoid; lepromatous is worse (failed cell-mediated immunity), tuberculoid is self-limited.

Rickettsiae

Rickettsiae are obligate intracellular parasites (except *R. quintana*) and need CoA and NAD. All except *Coxiella* are transmitted by an arthropod vector and cause headache, fever, and rash; *Coxiella* is an atypical rickettsia, since it is transmitted by aerosol. Tetracycline is the treatment of choice for most rickettsial infections.

Classic triad: headache, fever, rash (vasculitis)

Lyme disease

Classic symptom is erythema chronicum migrans, an expanding red rash. Also affects joints, CNS, and heart. Caused by *Borrelia burgdorferi,* which is transmitted by the tick *Ixodes.*

Mice and deer are important reservoirs.

Treat with tetracycline.

3 stages of Lyme disease:

Stage 1: Erythema chronicum migrans, flu-like symptoms

Stage 2: Neurologic and cardiac manifestations

Stage 3: Autoimmune migratory polyarthritis

Rickettsial diseases and vectors

Rocky Mountain spotted fever (tick): *Rickettsia rickettsii.*

Endemic typhus (fleas): *R. typhi.*

Epidemic typhus (human body louse): *R. prowazekii.*

Scrub typhus (mite): *R. tsutsugamushi.*

Q fever (inhaled aerosols): *Coxiella burnetii.*

Treatment for all: tetracycline.

TyPHus has centriPHugal (outward) spread of rash, sPotted fever is centriPetal (inward). Q fever is Queer because it has no rash, has no vector, has negative Weil-Felix, and its causative organism can survive outside for long time and doesn't have *Rickettsia* as its genus name.

Rocky Mountain spotted fever

Caused by *Rickettsia rickettsii.*

Symptoms: rash on palms and soles (migrating to wrists, ankles, then trunk), headache, fever.

Endemic to East Coast (despite name).

Palm and sole rash is seen in Rocky Mountain spotted fever and syphilis.

Chlamydiae	Chlamydiae are obligate intracellular parasites that cause mucosal infections. Two forms: 1. Elementary body (small, dense), which enters cell via endocytosis 2. Initial or reticular body, which replicates in cell by fission ⊘Chlamydiae cause arthritis, conjunctivitis, and nongono-coccal urethritis. The peptidoglycan wall is unusual in that it lacks muramic acid. Treatment: erythromycin or tetracycline.	*Chlamys* = cloak (intracellular). *Chlamydia psittaci* notable for an avian reservoir. *C. trachomatis* only infects humans. Lab diagnosis: cytoplasmic inclusions seen on Giemsa or fluorescent-antibody stained smear.
Chlamydial serotypes	Types A, B, and C: chronic infection, causes blindness in Africa. Types D-K: urethritis/PID, neonatal pneumonia, or neonatal conjunctivitis. Types L1, L2, and L3: lymphogranuloma venereum (positive Frei test). TWAR = new strain, pneumonia. Now called *C. pneumoniae*.	**ABC = Africa/Blindness/Chronic** infection. **L1-3 = Lymphogranuloma** venereum. D-K = everything else. Neonatal disease acquired by passage through infected birth canal.
Spirochetes	The spirochetes are spiral-shaped bacteria with axial filaments and include *Borrelia* (big size), *Leptospira*, and *Treponema*. Only *Borrelia* can be visualized using aniline dyes (Wright's stain or Giemsa stain).	**BLT. B is big.** *Leptospira* = thin spiral.
Treponemal disease	Treponemes are spirochetes. *Treponema pallidum* causes syphilis. *T. pertenue* causes yaws (a tropical infection that is not an STD although VDRL test is positive).	
VDRL versus FTA-ABS	FTA-ABS is specific for treponemes, turns positive earliest in disease, and remains positive longest during disease. VDRL is less specific.	FTA-**ABS** = FTA-**ABS**olute: 1. Most specific 2. Earliest positive 3. Remains positive the longest
VDRL false positives	VDRL detects nonspecific Ab that reacts with beef cardiolipin. Used for diagnosis of syphilis, but many biological false positives, including viral infection (mononucleosis, hepatitis), some drugs, rheumatic fever, rheumatoid arthritis, SLE, and leprosy.	**VDRL** = **V**enereal **D**isease (also **V**ery **D**oubtful) **R**esearch **L**aboratory. The **3 As** of false positives: **A**ged, **A**ddiction, **A**utoimmune.

Mycoplasma
pneumoniae

Mycoplasma pneumoniae is classic cause of atypical "walking" pneumonia (insidious onset, headache, non-productive cough). High titer of cold agglutinins. Grown on Eaton's agar.
Treatment: tetracycline or erythromycin (bugs are penicillin resistant because they have no cell wall).

No cell wall.
Only bacterial membrane containing cholesterol.
Mycoplasma pneumonia is less frequent in patients over age 30.
Frequent outbreaks in military recruits and prisons.

Candida albicans

Systemic or superficial fungal infection (budding yeast with pseudohyphae, germ tube formation at 37 °C). Thrush in throat with immunocompromised patients (neonates, steroids, diabetes, AIDS), endocarditis in IV drug users, vaginitis, diaper rash.
Treatment: nystatin for superficial infection; ampho-tericin B for serious systemic infection.

Alba = white.

Systemic mycoses

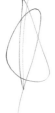

Disease	Endemic location	Notes
Coccidioidomycosis	Southwestern USA	San Joaquin Valley or desert (desert bumps)
Histoplasmosis	Mississippi and Ohio River valleys	Bird or bat droppings
Blastomycosis	States east of Mississippi River and Central America	Big, Broad-Based Budding
Paracoccidioidomy-cosis	Rural Latin America	"Captain's wheel" appearance

All of the above are dimorphic fungi, which are mold in soil (at lower temperature) and yeast in tissue (at higher/body temperature: 37 °C) except coccidioidomycosis, which is a spherule in tissue.

Cold = Mold
Culture on Sabouraud's agar.

Opportunistic fungal infections

Candida albicans	Thrush in immunocompromised (neonates, steroids, diabetes, AIDS), vulvovaginitis (high pH, diabetes, use of antibiotics), disseminated candidiasis (to any organ), chronic mucocutaneous candidiasis.
Aspergillus fumigatus	Ear fungus, lung cavity aspergilloma ("fungus ball"), invasive aspergillosis. **Mold** with septate hyphae that branch at a V-shaped (45°) angle. Not dimorphic.
Cryptococcus neoformans	Cryptococcal meningitis, cryptococcosis. Heavily encapsulated **yeast**. Not dimorphic. Found in soil, pigeon droppings. Culture of Sabouraud's agar. Stains with India ink. Latex agglutination test detects polysaccharide capsular antigen.
Mucor and *Rhizopus* species	Mucormycosis. **Mold** with irregular nonseptate hyphae branching at wide angles (≥ 90°). Disease mostly in ketoacidotic diabetic and leukemic patients.

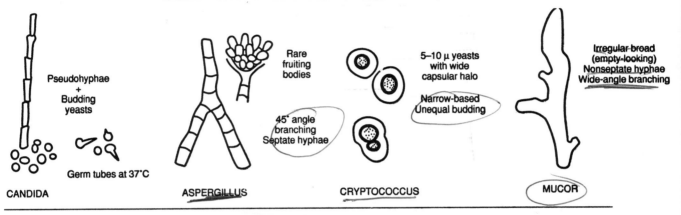

Pneumocystis carinii **(PCP)**	Causes pneumonia. Yeast (originally classified as protozoan). Inhaled. Most infections asymptomatic. Immunosuppression (e.g., AIDS) predisposes to disease. Silver stain of lung tissue. Treat with TMP-SMX.

Sporothrix schenckii

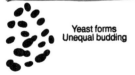

Yeast forms
Unequal budding

Sporotrichosis. Dimorphic fungus that lives on vegetation. When traumatically introduced into the skin, typically by a thorn ("rose gardener's" disease), causes local pustule or ulcer with nodules along draining lymphatics. Little systemic illness. Cigar-shaped budding cells visible in pus.

Encapsulated bacteria	Examples are *Streptococcus pneumoniae* (also known as pneumococcus), *Hemophilus influenzae* (especially B serotype), *Neisseria meningitidis* (also known as meningococcus), and *Klebsiella pneumoniae*. Polysaccharide capsule is an antiphagocytic virulence factor. Positive **Quellung** reaction: if encapsulated bug is present, capsule **swells** when specific anticapsular antisera are added.	IgG$_2$ necessary for immune response. Capsule serves as antigen in vaccines (Pneumovax, H. influenzae B, meningococcal vaccines). **Quellung** = capsular "swellung."

Normal flora: dominant

Skin–*S. epidermidis*
Nose–*S. aureus*
Oropharynx–Viridans streptococci
Dental plaque–*S. mutans*
Colon–*B. fragilis* > *E. coli*
Vagina–*Lactobacillus, E. coli,* group B strep

Neonates delivered by cesarean section have no flora, but are rapidly colonized after birth.

Lower respiratory tract infections

Leading bugs by age group:
Neonates: *E. coli,* group B strep
Infants: *Chlamydia* and RSV
Children: viruses
Teens: *Mycoplasma*
Adults: pneumococci

Neonates get infected with vaginal flora when delivered vaginally.

Meningitis: bacterial

Infants (birth to 6 wk): Group B strep, *E. coli, Listeria monocytogenes*
Children (6 mo–3 yrs): *H. influenzae*
Young adults (3–15 yrs): *N. meningitidis*
Adults (> 15 yrs): *S. pneumoniae*

Brain, an encapsulated (skull) organ, is infected by encapsulated bugs.

Meningitis: nonbacterial

Viral meningitis is often caused by the nonpolio enteroviruses, which are classified as picornaviruses: echovirus, coxsackievirus. Ninety percent of all viral meningitis occurs in those under age 30. Fungal meningitis is often caused by *Cryptococcus neoformans.*

Cryptomeningitis associated with pigeon droppings. *C. neoformans* stains with India ink.

CSF findings

Bacterial: pressure ↑, polys ↑, proteins ↑, sugar ↓.
Viral: pressure normal/↑, lymphs ↑, proteins **normal,** sugar **normal.**
TB/fungal: pressure ↑, lymphs ↑, proteins ↑, sugar ↓.

Osteomyelitis

Most people: *S. aureus*
Sexually active: *N. gonorrhoeae*
Drug addicts: *Pseudomonas aeruginosa*
Sickle cell: *Salmonella*
Hip replacement: *S. aureus* and *S. epidermidis*

Assume *S. aureus* if no other information.
Most osteomyelitis occurs in children.

Urinary tract infections

Ambulatory: *E. coli* (50–80%), *Klebsiella* (8–10%). *Staphylococcus saprophyticus* (10–30%) is the second most common cause of UTI in young ambulatory women.
Hospital: *E. coli, Proteus, Klebsiella, Serratia, Pseudomonas.*
Epidemiology: women to men = 30 to 1 (short urethra colonized by fecal flora).

UTIs mostly caused by ascending infections. In males: babies with congenital defects; elderly with enlarged prostates.

Pelvic inflammatory disease	Top bugs: *Chlamydia trachomatis* (subacute, often undiagnosed), *N. gonorrhoeae* (acute, high fever). *C. trachomatis* is the most common STD in the US (3–4 million cases per year). PID may include salpingitis, endometritis, hydrosalpinx, and tubo-ovarian abscess.	Salpingitis is a risk factor for ectopic pregnancy, infertility, chronic pelvic pain, and adhesions.

Nosocomial infections	By risk factor: • Newborn nursery: CMV • Urinary catheterization: *E. coli, Proteus mirabilis* • Respiratory therapy equipment: *P. aeruginosa* • Work in renal dialysis unit: HBV • Hyperalimentation: *Candida albicans* • Water aerosols: *Legionella*	Presume *Pseudomonas air-uginosa* when air or burns are involved; *Legionella* when water source is involved. The two most common causes of nosocomial infections are *E. coli* (UTI) and *S. aureus* (wound infection).

Bug hints (if all else fails)	Pus, empyema, abscess: *S. aureus* Pediatric infection: *H. influenzae* Aerobic infection: *P. aeruginosa* • Branching rods in oral infection: *Actinomyces israelii*	Kids get the flu (*H. inFLUenza*).

Weil-Felix reaction	Weil-Felix reaction assays for antirickettsial antibodies, which cross-react with *Proteus* antigen. Weil-Felix is usually positive for typhus and Rocky Mountain spotted fever but negative for Q fever.

UTI bugs

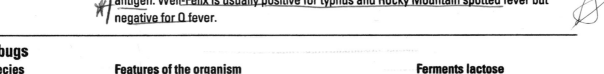

Species	Features of the organism	Ferments lactose
Escherichia coli	Colonies show metallic sheen on EMB agar	Yes
Enterobacter cloacae	Often nosocomial and drug-resistant	Yes
Klebsiella pneumoniae	Large mucoid capsule and viscous colonies	Yes
Serratia marcescens	Some strains produce a red pigment Often nosocomial and drug resistant	No
Proteus mirabilis	Motility causes "swarming" on agar Produces urease; associated with Struvite stones	No
Pseudomonas aeruginosa	Blue-green pigment and fruity odor Usually nosocomial and drug resistant	No

Special growth requirements

Bug	Media used for isolation	
H. influenzae	Chocolate agar with factors V (NAD) and X (hematin)	When a child has the flu, mom goes to the five (V) and dime (X) store to buy some chocolate.
N. gonorrhoeae	Thayer–Martin media	
B. pertussis	Bordet–Gengou (potato) agar	
C. diphtheriae	Tellurite agar	
M. tuberculosis	Löwenstein–Jensen agar	
S. aureus	Mannitol–salt agar	
M. pneumoniae	Eaton's agar	
Lactose-fermenting enterics (e.g., *Escherichia, Klebsiella,* and *Enterobacter*)	Pink colonies on MacConkey's agar	
Legionella pneumophila	Charcoal yeast extract agar buffered with ↑ iron and cysteine	
Fungi	Sabouraud's agar	

MICROBIOLOGY—VIRUSES

DNA viral strands	All DNA viruses except the Parvoviridae are dsDNA. All are linear except papovaviruses and hepadnaviruses (circular).	All are dsDNA (like our cells) except "part-of-a-virus" (parvovirus) is ssDNA.
RNA viral strands	All RNA viruses except Reoviridae are ssRNA.	All are ssRNA (like our mRNA) except "**re**peato-virus" (**Re**ovirus) is dsRNA.
Naked viral genome infectivity	Naked nucleic acids of most dsDNA (except poxviruses and HBV) and (+) strand ssRNA (≈mRNA) viruses are infectious. Naked nucleic acids of (−) strand ssRNA and dsRNA viruses are not infectious.	Viral nucleic acids with the same structure as host nucleic acids are infective alone; others require special enzymes (contained in intact virion).
Enveloped viruses	Generally, enveloped viruses acquire their envelopes from plasma membrane upon exit from cell. Exceptions are herpesviruses, which acquire envelopes from nuclear membrane.	
Virus ploidy	All viruses are haploid (with one copy of DNA or RNA) except retroviruses, which have two identical ssRNA molecules (≈diploid).	

Viral vaccines	• Live attenuated: measles, mumps, rubella, Sabin polio, VZV.	salK = Killed.
	• Killed: rabies, influenza, hepatitis A, and Salk polio vaccines.	MMR = Measles, Mumps, Rubella.
	• Recombinant: HBV (antigen = recombinant HBsAg).	

Viral replication

| DNA viruses: | All replicate in the nucleus (except pox virus). |
| RNA viruses: | All replicate in the cytoplasm (except influenza virus). |

Viral genetics

Recombination	Exchange of genes between 2 chromosomes by crossing over within regions of significant base sequence homology.
Reassortment	When viruses with segmented genomes (e.g., influenza virus) exchange segments. High-frequency recombination.
Complementation	When one of 2 viruses that infects the cell has a mutation that results in a nonfunctional protein. The nonmutated virus "complements" the mutated one by making a functional protein that serves both viruses.
Phenotypic mixing	Genome of virus A can be coated with the surface proteins of virus B. Type B protein coat determines the infectivity of the phenotypically mixed virus. However, the progeny from this infection has a type A coat; encoded by its type A genetic material.

| Viral vaccines: dead or alive | Live attenuated vaccines induce humoral and cell-mediated immunity, but have reverted to virulence on rare occasion. Killed vaccines induce only humoral immunity but are stable. | Dangerous to give live vaccines to immunocompromised patients or their close contacts. |

| Prions and slow viruses | Creutzfeldt-Jakob disease (CJD), kuru, SSPE (a late sequela of measles), PML (immunocompromised patients, owing to reactivation of JC virus or rarely SV40, papovaviruses), scrapie (sheep). | SSPE and PML have viral causes, whereas Creutzfeldt-Jakob disease and kuru are probably caused by prions. |

Hepatitis transmission

HAV (RNA virus) is transmitted primarily by fecal-oral route. Short incubation (3 weeks). No carriers.

Hep **A**: **A**symptomatic (usually)

HBV (DNA virus) is transmitted primarily by parenteral, sexual, and maternal-fetal routes. Long incubation (3 months). Carriers.

Hep **B**: **B**lood-borne

HCV is transmitted primarily via blood and resembles HBV in its course and severity. Carriers. Common cause of posttransfusion and IV drug use hepatitis in the United States.

Hep **C**: **C**hronic, **C**irrhosis, **C**arcinoma

HDV (delta agent) is a defective virus that requires HBs Ag as its envelope. Carriers.

Hep **D**: **D**efective, **D**ependent on HBV

HEV is transmitted enterically and causes water-borne epidemics. Resembles HAV in course, severity, incubation. High mortality rate in pregnant women. Both HBV and HCV predispose a patient to hepato-cellular carcinoma.

Hep **E**: **E**nteric

Microbiology

HIGH-YIELD FACTS

Hepatitis B serologic markers

	Description
IgM HAVAb	IgM antibody to HAV; best test to detect active hepatitis A.
HBsAg	Antigen found on surface of HBV; continued presence indicates carrier state.
HBsAb	Antibody to HBsAg; provides immunity to hepatitis B.
HBcAg	Antigen associated with core of HBV.
HBcAb	Antibody to HBcAg; positive during window phase. IgM HBcAb is an indicator of recent disease.
HBeAg	A second, different antigenic determinant in the HBV core. Important indicator of transmissibility.
HBeAb	Antibody to e antigen; indicates low transmissibility.

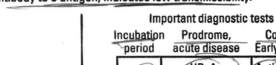

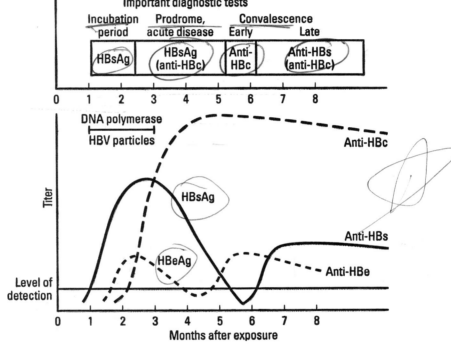

Months after exposure

Nonenveloped DNA viruses

Family	DNA structure	Important members
Adenovirus	DS (double stranded), linear	Adenovirus
Papovavirus	DS, circular	Papilloma virus
Parvovirus	SS (single stranded)	B19 virus

Enveloped DNA viruses

Family	DNA structure	Important members
Hepadnavirus	DS, incomplete circular	Hepatitis B virus
Herpesvirus	DS	HSV, CMV, EBV, VZV
Poxvirus	DS	Smallpox virus, vaccinia virus

Microbiology

HIGH-YIELD FACTS

Nonenveloped RNA viruses

Family	RNA structure	Important members
Calicivirus	SS, + polarity	Norwalk virus, hepatitis E virus
Picornavirus	SS, + polarity	Poliovirus, rhinovirus, hepatitis A virus, coxsackievirus, echovirus
Reovirus	DS 10 segments	Reovirus, rotavirus

Enveloped RNA viruses

Family	RNA structure	Important members
Flavivirus	SS, + polarity	Yellow fever, dengue, HCV
Orthomyxovirus	SS, − polarity, 8 segments	Influenza
Paramyxovirus	SS, − polarity, 1 piece	Measles, mumps, RSV, parainfluenza
Rhabdovirus	SS, − polarity, 1 piece	Rabies
Retrovirus	SS, + polarity, 2 copies	HIV, HTLV (causes leukemia)
Togavirus	SS, + polarity	Rubella

Segmented viruses

All are RNA viruses. They include arenaviruses, reoviruses, bunyaviruses, and orthomyxoviruses (influenza viruses). Influenza virus consists of 8 segments of negative stranded RNA. These segments can undergo reassortment, causing worldwide epidemics of the flu.

Arena = "grains of sand" (due to ribosomes in the viral capsid as seen on electron microscopy). **Reo** = **repeato** = segmented.

Picornavirus

Includes poliovirus, rhinovirus, coxsackievirus, echovirus, hepatitis A virus. RNA is translated into one large polypeptide which is cleaved by proteases into many small proteins. Can lead to aseptic meningitis (except rhinovirus and hep A virus).

The discovery of **polio**, on a **rhino** in **Coxsackie**, NY, was **echoed** around the world.

Rotavirus

Rotavirus, the agent of infantile gastroenteritis, is a segmented dsRNA virus (a reovirus).

ROTA = **R**ight **O**ut **T**he **A**nus.

Paramyxoviruses

Paramyxoviruses include those that cause parainfluenza (croup), mumps, and measles, as well as RSV, which causes respiratory tract infection in infants. Paramyxoviruses cause disease in children. All paramyxoviruses have 1 serotype.

Mumps virus

A paramyxovirus with one serotype. Symptoms: parotitis, orchitis (inflammation of testes), and aseptic meningitis. Can cause sterility.

Mumps gives you b**umps** (parotitis).

Measles virus

A paramyxovirus that causes measles. Koplik spots (bluish-gray spots on buccal mucosa) are diagnostic. SSPE, encephalitis (1 in 2000), or giant cell pneumonia (rarely, in immunosuppressed) are possible sequelae.

3 C's of measles:
Cough
Coryza
Conjunctivitis
Also look for Koplik spots.

Rabies virus	Negri bodies are characteristic cytoplasmic inclusions in neurons infected by rabies virus. Has bullet-shaped capsid. Rabies has long incubation period (weeks to 3 mo). Causes encephalitis with seizures and hydrophobia.	Rhabdovirus travels to the CNS by migrating in a retrograde fashion up nerve axons.
Arboviruses	Transmitted by arthropods (mosquitoes, ticks). Classic examples are dengue fever (also known as break-bone fever) and yellow fever. A variant of dengue fever in Southeast Asia is hemorrhagic shock syndrome.	
Yellow fever	Caused by flavivirus, an arbovirus transmitted by *Aedes* mosquitos. Virus has a monkey or human reservoir. Symptoms: high fever, black vomitus, and jaundice. Councilman bodies (acidophilic inclusions) may be seen in liver.	*Flavi* = yellow.
Mononucleosis	Caused by EBV, a herpesvirus. Characterized by fever, hepatosplenomegaly, pharyngitis, and lymphadenopathy (especially posterior auricular nodes). Peak incidence 15–20 y old. Positive heterophil Ab test. Abnormal circulating cytotoxic T cells (atypical lymphocytes).	Most common during peak kissing years.
Tzanck test	A smear of an opened skin vesicle to detect multi-nucleated giant cells. Used to assay for herpesvirus.	Tzanck heavens I don't have herpes.
Time course of HIV infection		

125

Opportunistic infections in AIDS

Bacterial	Tuberculosis, *M. avium-intracellulare* complex.	Alphabet soup: TB, MAC, HSV, VZV, CMV, PCP.
Viral	Herpes simplex, varicella-zoster virus, cytomegalovirus, progressive multifocal leukoencephalopathy (JC virus).	
Fungal	Thrush (*Candida albicans*), cryptococcosis (cryptococcal meningitis), histoplasmosis.	
Protozoal	Pneumocystis pneumonia, toxoplasmosis, cryptosporidiosis.	

Antibody structure

Variable part of L and H chains recognizes antigens. Constant part of H chain fixes IgM and IgG complement. Heavy chain contributes to Fc and Fab fractions. Light chain contributes only to Fab fraction.

Immunoglobulins

IgG	Opsonizes bacteria, fixes complement, neutralizes bacterial toxins and viruses, crosses the placenta.
IgA	Prevents attachment of bacteria and viruses to mucous membranes, does not fix complement. Monomer or dimer. Found in secretions.
IgM	Produced in the primary response to an antigen. Fixes complement but does not cross the placenta. Antigen receptor on the surface of B cells. Monomer or pentamer.
IgD	Unclear function. Found on the surface of many B cells and in serum.
IgE	Mediates immediate (type I) hypersensitivity by inducing the release of mediators from mast cells and basophils upon exposure to allergen. Mediates immunity to worms.

Ig epitopes

Allotype = Ig epitope common to a species.
Isotype = Ig epitope common to a single class of Ig (five classes, determined by heavy chain).
Idiotype = Ig epitope determined by antigen binding site.

Allotype = common to **ALL** in species.
Isotype = Iso (same). Common to same class.
Idiotype = Idiotypic (unique). Hypervariable region is unique.

Adjuvant definition

Adjuvants are nonspecific stimulators of the immune response but are not immunogenic by themselves. Adjuvants are given with a weak immunogen to enhance response.

Adjuvant = that which aids another.

MHC I and II	MHC = Major histocompatibility complex. Consists of 3 class I genes (A, B, C) and 3 class II genes (DP, DQ, DR). All nucleated cells have class I MHC proteins. Antigen-presenting cells (e.g., macrophages) also have class II MHC proteins. Class II are the main determinants of organ rejection.	Class I = 1 polypeptide, with β_2-microglobulin. Class II = 2 polypeptides, an α and a β chain.
T-cell glycoproteins	Helper T cells have CD4, which binds to class II MHC on antigen-presenting cells. Cytotoxic T cells have CD8, which binds to class I MHC on virus-infected cells.	Product of CD and MHC = 8. (CD4 $\times$ MHC II = 8 = CD8 $\times$ MHC I.)
Precipitin curve	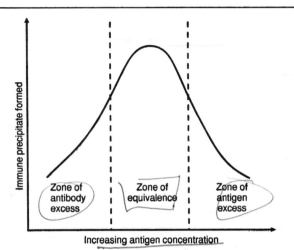	In the presence of a constant amount of antibody, the amount of immune precipitate formed is plotted as a function of increasing amounts of antigen.

Important cytokines

IL-1	Secreted by macrophages. Stimulates T cells, B cells, neutrophils, fibroblasts, epithelial cells to grow, differentiate, or synthesize specific products. Is an endogenous pyrogen.	"Hot T bone stEAk" IL-1: fever (**hot**) IL-2: stimulates **T** cells IL-3: stimulates **bone** marrow IL-4: stimulates Ig**E** production IL-5: stimulates Ig**A** production
IL-2	Secreted by helper T cells. Stimulates growth of helper and cytotoxic T cells.	
IL-3	Secreted by activated T cells. Supports the growth and differentiation of bone marrow stem cells. Has a function similar to GM-CSF.	
IL-4	Secreted by helper T cells. Promotes growth of B cells. Enhances the synthesis of IgE and IgG.	
IL-5	Secreted by helper T cells. Promotes differentiation of B cells. Enhances the synthesis of IgA. Stimulates production and activation of eosinophils.	
Gamma interferon	Secreted by helper T cells. Stimulates macrophages.	

Complement

Complement defends against gram-negative bacteria. Activated by IgG or IgM in the classic pathway, and activated by toxins (including endotoxin), aggregated IgA, or other conditions in the alternate pathway.

C1, C2, C3, C4: viral neutralization.
C3b: opsonization.
C3a, C5a: anaphylaxis.
C5a: neutrophil chemotaxis.
C5b-9: cytolysis by membrane attack complex (MAC) (deficiency in *Neisseria* sepsis).
Deficiency of C1 esterase inhibitor leads to angioedema (overactive complement).

Alternative

Microbial surfaces (nonspecific activators) ⟶ C3(H$_2$O) + B + D ⟶ $\overline{\text{C3b,Bb}}$ (C3 convertase)

C3 ⟶ $\overline{\text{C3b,Bb,C3b}}$ + C3a (C5 convertase)

Target cell membrane (M)

C5 ⟶ C5a + MC5b ⟶ MC5b,6,7 ⟶ MC5b,6,7,8,9 (membrane attack complex) ⟶ LYSIS, CYTOTOXICITY

C7   C9
C6   C8

C3 ⟶ C3a + $\overline{\text{C4b,2b,3b}}$ (C5 convertase)

Classic

Antigen-antibody complexes ⟶ C1 ⟶ $\overline{\text{C1}}$ ⟶ C2, C4 ⟶ $\overline{\text{C4b,2b}}$ (C3 convertase)

Interferon mechanism

Interferons are proteins that place uninfected cells in an antiviral state. Interferons induce the production of a second protein that inhibits viral protein synthesis by degrading viral mRNA (but not host mRNA).

Interferes with viral protein synthesis.

Hypersensitivity

Type I	**Anaphylactic and atopic:** Ag cross-links IgE on presensitized mast cells and basophils, triggering release of vasoactive amines. Reaction develops rapidly after Ag exposure due to preformed Ab. Possible manifestations include anaphylaxis, asthma, or local wheal and flare.	First and fast (anaphylaxis). I, II, and III are all antibody mediated.
Type II	**Cytotoxic:** IgM, IgG bind to Ag on "enemy" cell, leading to lysis (by complement) or phagocytosis. Examples include autoimmune hemolytic anemia, Rh disease (erythroblastosis fetalis), Goodpasture's syndrome.	Cy-**2**-toxic. Antibody and complement mediated.
Type III	**Immune complex:** Ag-Ab complexes activate complement, which attracts neutrophils; neutrophils release lysosomal enzymes (e.g., PAN, immune complex GN).	Imagine an immune complex as **three** things stuck together: Ag–Ab–complement.
	Serum sickness is an immune complex disease (type III) in which Abs to the foreign proteins are produced (takes 5 days). Immune complexes form and are deposited in membranes, where they fix complement (leads to tissue damage). More common than Arthus reaction.	Most serum sickness is now caused by drugs (not serum).
	Arthus reaction is a local subacute Ab-mediated hypersensitivity (type III) reaction. Intradermal injection of Ag induces antibodies, which form Ag-Ab complexes in the skin. Characterized by edema, necrosis, and activation of complement.	Ag-Ab complexes cause the Arthus reaction.
Type IV	**Delayed (cell-mediated) type:** Sensitized T lymphocytes encounter antigen and then release lymphokines (leads to macrophage activation). Examples include TB skin test, transplant rejection, contact dermatitis.	4th and last = delayed. Cell mediated; therefore, it is not transferable by serum. **ACID** = **A**naphylactic and **A**topic (type I), **C**ytotoxic (type II), **I**mmune complex (type III), **D**elayed (cell-mediated) (type IV).

Passive versus active immunity

Passive:	Based on receiving preformed antibodies from another host. Rapid onset. Short life span of antibodies.	After exposure to tetanus toxin or botulinum toxin patients are given preformed antibodies (passive) for rapid availability of protection.
Active:	Induced after exposure with foreign antigens. Slow onset. Long-lasting protection.	

Immune deficiencies

Thymic aplasia (DiGeorge's syndrome)	T-cell deficiency. Thymus and parathyroids fail to develop owing to failure of development of the 3rd and 4th pharyngeal pouches. Presents with tetany owing to hypocalcemia.
Severe combined immunodeficiency	B- and T-cell deficiency. Defect in early stem-cell differentiation. Presents with recurrent viral, bacterial, fungal, and protozoal infections. May have multiple causes, e.g., failure to synthesize class II MHC antigens, defective IL-2 receptors, or adenosine deaminase deficiency.
Wiskott–Aldrich syndrome	B- and T-cell deficiency. Defect in the ability to mount an IgM response to capsular poly-saccharides of bacteria. Associated with elevated IgA levels, normal IgE levels, and low IgM levels. Triad of symptoms includes recurrent pyogenic infections, eczema, and thrombocytopenia.
Chronic granulomatous disease	Phagocyte deficiency. Defect in phagocytosis of neutrophils owing to lack of NADPH oxidase activity or similar enzymes. Presents with marked susceptibility to opportunistic infections with bacteria, especially *S. aureus*, and *Aspergillus*.
Chédiak–Higashi disease	Autosomal recessive defect in phagocytosis that results from microtubular and lysosomal defects of phagocytic cells. Presents with recurrent pyogenic infections by staphylococci and streptococci.
Job's syndrome	Neutrophils fail to respond to chemotactic stimuli. Associated with high levels of IgE. Presents with recurrent cold staphylococcal abscesses.
Bruton's agammaglobulinemia	B-cell deficiency. X-linked recessive defect associated with low levels of all classes of immunoglobulins. Associated with recurrent bacterial infections after 6 months of age, when levels of maternal IgG antibody decline.
Selective immunoglobulin deficiency	Deficiency in a specific class of immunoglobulins. Possibly due to a defect in isotype switching. Selective IgA deficiency is the most common selective immunoglobulin deficiency.
Ataxia–telangiectasia	B- and T-cell deficiency, with associated IgA deficiency. Presents with cerebellar problems (ataxia) and spider angiomas (telangiectasia).

Transplant rejection

Hyperacute rejection—Antibody mediated due to the presence of preformed anti-donor antibodies in the transplant recipient. Occurs within minutes after transplantation. Type II cytotoxic reaction (localized Arthus reaction). Irreversible.

Acute rejection—Cell mediated due to cytotoxic T lymphocytes reacting against foreign MHCs. Occurs weeks after transplantation. Reversible with immunosuppressants such as cyclosporin and OKT3.

Chronic rejection—Antibody-mediated vascular damage (fibrinoid necrosis); occurs months to years after transplantation. Irreversible.

Microbiology

1. Principles and interpretation of bacteriological lab tests (cultures, incubation time, drug sensitivities, specific growth requirements).
2. Distinguishing features of staphylococci (coagulase, antibiotic sensitivity, etc.).
3. Distinguishing features of streptococci (hemolysis, antibiotic sensitivity, etc.).
4. Complications of streptococcal infection (e.g., acute glomerulonephritis, rheumatic fever).
5. Dermatologic manifestations of bacterial infection (e.g., syphilis, Rocky Mountain spotted fever, meningococcemia).
6. Modes of transmission of the common sexually transmitted diseases (e.g., syphilis, AIDS, herpes).
7. Diagnostic testing for STDs (e.g., syphilis, HIV).
8. Tick-transmitted infections (e.g., Lyme disease).
9. Microbiology and pathology of prion diseases (e.g., Creutzfeldt-Jakob disease, scrapie).
10. Infectious causes of food poisoning.
11. Viral gastroenteritis in children versus adults.
12. Common infections leading to pneumonia.
13. Causes and clinical features of pelvic inflammatory disease.
14. Infections that cause *in utero* birth defects (e.g., ToRCH—toxoplasmosis, rubella, CMV, herpes).
15. Common nosocomial infections (e.g., *Pseudomonas, Klebsiella*).

Immunology

1. Principles and interpretation of immunologic tests (e.g., enzyme-linked immunosorbent assay, Coombs' test, Ouchterlony reactions, complement fixation).
2. Specifics of immune complex–related diseases (e.g., Goodpasture's syndrome, systemic lupus erythematosus, rheumatoid arthritis).
3. Genetic mechanisms involved in immunoglobulin diversity and class switching (e.g., IgM to IgG).
4. Mechanisms of congenital and acquired immunodeficiencies.
5. Mechanisms of antigenic variation in bacteria and parasites.

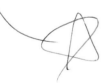

Pathology

Questions dealing with this discipline are difficult to prepare for because of the sheer volume of material. Review the basic principles and hallmark characteristics of the disease. Given the clinical orientation of the Step 1, it is no longer enough to know the "trigger words" or key associations of certain diseases (eg, café au lait macules and neurofibromatosis); you must also know the clinical descriptions of these trigger words. Learn the diseases that are the most common causes of various clinical conditions (e.g., the most common primary brain tumor in adults). With the new clinical slant of the USMLE Step 1, it is also important to review the classic presenting signs and symptoms of diseases as well as their associated laboratory findings. The examination includes a number of color photomicrographs and photographs of gross specimens, which are shown in the setting of a brief clinical history. However, read the question and the choices carefully before looking at the illustration, since the history alone is usually sufficient to identify the pathologic process. Pay attention to potential clues such as age, sex, ethnicity, and activity.

Congenital
Neoplastic
Gastrointestinal
Neurologic
Rheumatic/
Autoimmune
Vascular/Cardiac
Other
Findings
High-Yield Topics

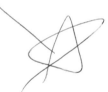

Pathology

HIGH-YIELD FACTS

Common malformations

1. Heart defects
2. Hypospadias
3. Cleft lip with or without cleft palate
4. Congenital hip dislocation
5. Spina bifida
6. Anencephaly
7. Pyloric stenosis (associated with polyhydramnios)

Both spina bifida and anencephaly are associated with increased levels of AFP in the amniotic fluid and maternal serum.

Congenital heart disease

R-to-L shunts (early cyanosis)

1. Tetralogy of Fallot (most common cause of early cyanosis)
2. Transposition of great arteries
3. Truncus arteriosus
4. Tricuspid atresia
5. Total anomalous pulmonary return

The 5 T's:
Tetralogy
Transposition
Truncus
Tricuspid
Total

L-to-R shunts (late cyanosis)

1. VSD (most common congenital cardiac anomaly)
2. ASD
3. PDA

Frequency: VSD > ASD > PDA.
↑ pulmonary resistance due to arteriolar thickening
→ progressive pulmonary hypertension

Tetralogy of Fallot

1. Pulmonary stenosis
2. VSD
3. RVH
4. Large aorta overriding the VSD

This leads to early cyanosis from a R-to-L shunt across the VSD. On x-ray, boot-shaped heart due to RVH.

Think of pulmonary outflow stenosis/atresia as primary event with VSD and RVH as immediate consequences and with right-sided aorta as chronic compensation.
Tetra = 4.

Transposition of great vessels

Aorta leaves RV (anterior) and pulmonary trunk leaves LV (posterior) → separation of systemic and pulmonary circulations. Not compatible with life unless a shunt is present to allow adequate mixing of blood (e.g., VSD, PDA, or patent foramen ovale).

Without surgical correction, most infants die within the first months of life. Common in offspring of diabetic mothers.

Coarctation of aorta

Infantile type: aortic stenosis proximal to insertion of ductus arteriosus (preductal).
Adult type: stenosis is distal to ductus arteriosus (postductal). Associated with notching of the ribs, hypertension in upper extremities, weak pulses in lower extremities.

Affects males:females 3:1.
Check femoral pulses on physical exam. The **IN**fantile type is **IN** close to the heart; a**D**ult type is **D**istal to **D**uctus.
Infantile type is associated with Turner's syndrome.

Patent ductus arteriosus	In fetal period, shunt is R-to-L (normal). In neonatal period, lung resistance decreases and shunt becomes L-to-R with subsequent RV hypertrophy and failure (abnormal). Associated with a continuous, "machine-like" murmur. Patency is maintained by PGE synthesis and low oxygen tension.	Indomethacin is used to close a PDA. PGE is used to keep a PDA open, which may be necessary in conditions such as transposition of the great vessels.
Eisenmenger's complex	Late cyanotic shunt (R → L) due to pulmonary hypertension and RV hypertrophy from a long-standing VSD, ASD, or PDA.

Autosomal trisomies

Down's syndrome (trisomy 21), 1:700	Most common chromosomal disorder and cause of hereditary mental retardation. Findings: mental retardation, flat facial profile, prominent epicanthal folds, **duodenal atresia** (double bubble sign on x-ray), congenital heart disease (most common malformation is **endocardial cushion defect**), **Alzheimer's disease** in affected individuals > 35 years old, associated with an increased risk of ALL. 95% of cases are due to meiotic nondisjunction of homologous chromosomes, 5% of cases are due to Robertsonian translocation. Associated with advanced maternal age.
Edwards' syndrome (trisomy 18), 1:8000	Findings: severe mental retardation, **rocker bottom feet**, low-set ears, **micrognathia**, congenital heart disease, clenched hands (flexion of fingers), prominent occiput. Death usually occurs within 1 year of birth.
Patau's syndrome (trisomy 13), 1:6000	Findings: severe mental retardation, **microphthalmia**, microcephaly, cleft lip/palate, abnormal forebrain structures, polydactyly, congenital heart disease. Death usually occurs within 1 year of birth.

Genetic gender disorders

Klinefelter's syndrome [male] (XXY), 1:850	Testicular atrophy, eunuchoid body shape, tall, gynecomastia, female distribution of hair.	One of the most common causes of hypogonadism in males.
Turner's syndrome [female] (XO), 1:3000	Short stature, ovarian dysgenesis, webbing of neck secondary to cystic hygroma, coarctation of the aorta.	Imagine **turn**ing into a circle (XO).
Double Y males [male] (XYY), 1:1000	Phenotypically normal, very tall, severe acne, antisocial behavior.	Observed with increased frequency among inmates of penal institutions.

Pseudohermaphrodite

	Disagreement between the phenotypic and gonadal sex.
Female pseudo-hermaphrodite (XX)	Ovaries present, but external genitalia are virilized or ambiguous. Due to excessive and inappropriate exposure to androgenic steroids during early gestation (ie, congenital adrenal hyperplasia or exogenous administration of androgens during pregnancy).
Male pseudo-hermaphrodite (XY)	Testes present, but external genitalia are female or ambiguous. Most common form is testicular feminization, which results from a mutation in the androgen receptor gene and is X-linked recessive.

Cri-du-chat syndrome

Congenital deletion of short arm of chromosome 5 (46 XX or XY, 5p–).
Findings: microcephaly, severe mental retardation, **high-pitched crying/mewing**, epicanthal folds, cardiac abnormalities.

Cri-du-chat = cry of the cat.

Fragile X syndrome

X-linked recessive defect. It is the second most common cause of hereditary mental retardation (the most common cause is Down's syndrome). Associated with macro-orchidism (enlarged testes), long face with a large jaw, and large everted ears.

DiGeorge's syndrome

Due to failure of development of 3rd + 4th pharyngeal pouches and associated with:
1. Total absence of cell-mediated immune responses (lack of thymus)
2. Tetany (lack of parathyroids and hence hypocalcemia)
3. Congenital defects of heart and great vessels

Think "deep gorge" where thymus should have been. Recurrent viral and fungal infections.

Duchenne's muscular dystrophy

An X-linked recessive muscular disease featuring a defective dystrophin gene, leading to accelerated muscle breakdown. Onset before 5 years of age. Weakness begins in pelvic girdle muscles and progresses superiorly. Pseudohypertrophy of calf muscles due to fibro-fatty replacement of muscle; cardiac myopathy. The use of Gower's maneuver, requiring assistance of the upper extremities to stand up, is characteristic but not specific (indicates proximal lower limb weakness).

Cystic fibrosis

Autosomal recessive defect in CFTR gene on chromosome 7. Defective Cl– channel → secretion of abnormally thick mucus that plugs lungs, pancreas, salivary glands, and liver → recurrent pulmonary infections (*Pseudomonas aeruginosa* and *Staphylococcus aureus*), chronic bronchitis, bronchiectasis, malabsorption and steatorrhea, meconium ileus in newborns. Increased concentration of Cl– ions in sweat (diagnostic).

Infertility in males. Fat-soluble vitamin deficiencies (A, D, K).

Childhood polycystic kidney disease

Autosomal recessive bilateral enlargement of kidneys, with numerous small cysts of collecting ducts at right angles to the cortical surface. Associated with multiple liver cysts, congenital hepatic fibrosis, and proliferation of bile ducts.

Autosomal dominant diseases

Adult polycystic kidney disease	Bilateral massive enlargement of kidneys due to multiple large cysts. Patients present with pain, hematuria, hypertension, progresive renal failure. Associated with polycystic liver disease, berry aneurysms, mitral valve prolapse.
Familial hypercholesterolemia	Elevated LDL owing to defective or absent LDL receptor. Heterozygotes (1 in 500) have cholesterol ≈ 300 mg/dL. Homozygotes (very rare) have cholesterol ≈ 700+ mg/dL, severe atherosclerotic disease early in life and tendon xanthomas (classically in the Achilles tendon). Myocardial infarction may develop before age 20.
Marfan's syndrome	Fibrillin gene mutation → connective tissue disorders. Skeletal abnormalities: Tall with long extremities, hyperextensive joints, and long, tapering fingers and toes. Cardiovascular: Cystic medial necrosis of aorta → aortic incompetence and dissecting aortic aneurysms. Floppy mitral valve. Ocular: Subluxation of lenses.
Von Recklinghausen's disease (NFT1)	Findings: café au lait spots, neural tumors, Lisch nodules (pigmented iris hamartomas). On long arm of chromosome 17; 17 letters in Von Recklinghausen.
Von Hippel-Lindau disease	Findings: hemangioblastomas of retina/cerebellum/medulla; about half of affected individuals develop multiple bilateral renal cell carcinomas and other tumors. Associated with deletion of short arm of chromosome 3 (3p).
Huntington's disease	Findings: depression, progressive dementia, choreiform movements, caudate atrophy and decreased levels of GABA and acetylcholine in the brain. Symptoms manifest in affected individuals between the ages of 20 and 50. Gene located on chromosome 4.
Familial polyposis coli	Colon becomes covered with adenomatous polyps after puberty; unless the colon is removed, the risk of cancer is 100%. Deletion of APC gene on chromosome 5.

Congenital CNS defects

Spina bifida: failure of bony spinal canal to close but no structural herniation. Usually seen at lower vertebral levels. Associated with low folic acid intake during pregnancy.

Meningocele: meninges herniate through spinal canal defect.

Meningomyelocele: meninges and spinal cord herniate through spinal canal defect.

Teratogens

Examples include actinomycin D (preimplantation), x-rays, iodine, thalidomide, aminopterin, DES, alcohol, warfarin, phenytoin, retinoic acid (Accutane). 3rd–8th week of pregnancy most susceptible.

Note that teratogens can act before pregnancy is discovered. Fetal infections can also cause malformations.

Pathology *(side tab)*

HIGH-YIELD FACTS *(side tab)*

Blood dyscrasias

Sickle cell anemia	Single amino acid replacement in β-chain (substitution of normal glutamic acid with valine). Low O_2 precipitates sickling. Heterozygotes are relatively malaria resistant (balanced polymorphism). Complications include aplastic crisis, autosplenectomy, ↑risk of encapsulated organism infection, salmonella osteomyelitis, and painful crisis (vaso-occlusive).	8% of American blacks carry the SC trait. 0.2% have the disease. Sickled cells are crescent-shaped RBCs. Average RBC survival in SC anemia is ≈ 120 days.
α-thalassemia	There are four α-globin genes. In α-thalassemia, the α-globin chain is underproduced (as a function of number of bad genes, one to four). There is no compensatory increase of any other chains. Hb Barts (γ_4-tetramers) or hydrops fetalis = no functional α-globin chains and intrauterine fetal death.	Thalassemia is prevalent in Mediterranean populations (*thalassa* = sea). Think of thala**SEA**mia.
β-thalassemia	In β-minor thalassemia (heterozygote), the β-chain is underproduced; in β-major (homozygote), the β-chain is absent. In both cases, fetal hemoglobin production is compensatorily increased but is inadequate.	β-thalassemia major results in severe anemia requiring blood transfusions. Cardiac failure due to secondary hemochromatosis.

HLA associations

	Disease
HLA-B27	Ankylosing spondylitis; Reiter's syndrome; postgonococcal arthritis
HLA-DR4	Rheumatoid arthritis
HLA-DR3	Sjögren's syndrome; chronic active hepatitis
HLA-DR2, HLA-DR3	Systemic lupus erythematosus
HLA-A3	Primary hemochromatosis

PATHOLOGY—NEOPLASTIC

Plasia definitions

Hyperplasia = Increase in number of cells (reversible).

Metaplasia = One adult cell type is replaced by another (reversible).

Dysplasia = An abnormal growth with loss of cellular orientation, shape, and size in comparison to normal tissue maturation, commonly preneoplastic (reversible).

Anaplasia = Abnormal cells lacking differentiation; like primitive cells of same tissue, often equated with undifferentiated malignant neoplasms. Tumor giant cells may be formed.

Neoplasia = Uncontrolled and excessive proliferation of cells. May be benign or malignant.

Precancerous conditions and associated malignancies	Condition	Neoplasm
	1. Down's syndrome	1. Acute lymphoblastic leukemia *ALL*
	2. Xeroderma pigmentosum	2. Squamous cell and basal cell carcinomas of skin
	3. Chronic atrophic gastritis, pernicious anemia, postsurgical gastric remnants	3. Gastric adenocarcinoma
	4. Tuberous sclerosis	4. Cerebral gliomas and cardiac rhabdomyomas
	5. Café au lait skin patches	5. Neurofibromatosis I
	6. Actinic keratosis	6. Squamous cell carcinoma of skin
	7. Barrett's esophagus	7. Esophageal adenocarcinoma
	8. Plummer–Vinson syndrome (atrophic glossitis, esophageal webs, plus anemia)	8. Squamous cell carcinoma of esophagus
	9. Cirrhosis (alcoholic, hepatitis B/C)	9. Hepatocellular carcinoma
	10. Ulcerative colitis	10. Colonic adenocarcinoma
	11. Paget's disease of bone	11. Secondary osteosarcoma and fibrosarcoma
	12. Immunodeficiency states	12. Malignant lymphomas
	13. AIDS	13. Aggressive B-cell lymphomas and Kaposi's sarcoma
	14. Autoimmune diseases (e.g., Hashimoto's thyroiditis, myasthenia gravis)	14. Malignant lymphoma (e.g., thyroid lymphoma), thymoma

Oncogenes	Associated tumor
myc	Burkitt's lymphoma
N-myc	Neuroblastoma
L-myc	Small cell carcinoma of lung
bcl-2	Follicular and undifferentiated lymphomas
erb-B2	Breast, ovarian, and gastric carcinomas

Tumor suppressor genes	Gene	Chromosome	Associated tumor
	APC	5q	Familial adenomatous polyposis coli, colorectal carcinoma
	WT-1	11p	Wilms' tumor
	Rb	13q	Retinoblastoma, osteosarcoma
	BRCA-2	13q	Breast cancer
	p53	17p	Most human cancers
	NF-1	17q	Neurofibromatosis type I
	BRCA-1	17q	Breast cancer, ovarian cancer
	DCC	18q	Carcinomas of colon and stomach
	NF-2	22q	Neurofibromatosis type II (acoustic neuroma)

Tumor markers

PSA, prostatic acid phosphatase	Prostatic carcinoma.
CEA	Carcinoembryonic antigen. Very nonspecific but produced by ~70% of colorectal and pancreatic cancers; also in gastric and breast carcinomas.
α-fetoprotein	Normally made by fetus. Hepatocellular carcinomas. Nonseminomatous germ cell tumors of the testis (e.g., yolk sac tumor).
β-hCG	Gestational trophoblastic tumors, hydatidiform moles, and choriocarcinomas. Useful as marker of tumor burden.
α_1-antitrypsin	Liver and yolk sac tumors.
CA-125	Ovarian tumors.
S-100	Melanoma, neural tumors, astrocytomas.
Bombesin	Neuroblastoma, small cell carcinomas, gastric and pancreatic carcinomas.

Enzyme markers

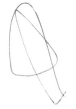

Serum enzyme	Major diagnostic use
Aminotransferases (AST and ALT)	Myocardial infarction (AST only) Viral hepatitis (ALT > AST) Alcoholic hepatitis (AST > ALT)
Amylase	Acute pancreatitis, mumps
Ceruloplasmin (decreased)	Wilson's disease
CPK (creatine phosphokinase)	Muscle disorders (e.g., DMD) and myocardial infarction (CPK-MB)
γ-glutamyl transpeptidase	Various liver diseases
LDH-1 (lactate dehydrogenase fraction 1)	Myocardial infarction (LDH1 > LDH2)
Lipase	Acute pancreatitis

Oncogenic viruses

	Associated cancer
HTLV-1	Adult T-cell leukemia
HBV	Hepatocellular carcinoma
EBV	Burkitt's lymphoma, nasopharyngeal carcinoma
HPV	Cervical carcinoma
Kaposi's sarcoma-associated herpesvirus (KSHV)	Kaposi's sarcoma

Pathology

HIGH-YIELD FACTS

Brain tumors

Adult — 70% above tentorium (e.g., cerebral hemispheres). Incidence: metastases > astrocytoma (including glioblastoma) > meningioma > pituitary tumor.

Childhood — 70% below tentorium (e.g., cerebellum). Second most common childhood neoplasm after leukemia. Incidence: medulloblastoma > astrocytoma > ependymoma.

Adults are taller than kids; therefore their tumors are supratentorial. Glioblastoma multiforme: necrosis and pseudopalisading; "butterfly" glioma.

Cardiac tumors

Myxomas are the most common 1° cardiac tumor in adults. 90% occur in the atria (mostly LA). Myxomas are usually described as a "ball-valve" obstruction in the LA. Rhabdomyomas are the most frequent 1° cardiac tumor in children.

Colorectal cancer risk factors

Risk factors for carcinoma of colon: colorectal villous adenomas, chronic inflammatory bowel disease, low-fiber diet, increasing age, familial polyposis, personal and family history of colon cancer.

Barrett's esophagus

Glandular (columnar epithelial) metaplasia—replacement of stratified squamous epithelium with gastric (columnar) epithelium in the distal esophagus. Predisposes to esophageal adenocarcinoma; usually secondary to gastroesophageal reflux.

Multiple endocrine neoplasias (MEN)

MEN Type I (Werner's syndrome)—Pancreas (e.g., ZE syndrome, insulinomas, VIPomas), parathyroid, and pituitary tumors. [adrenal + thyroid]

MEN Type IIa (Sipple's syndrome)— Medullary carcinoma of the thyroid, pheochromocytoma, parathyroid tumor or adenoma. PTP

MEN Type III (formerly MEN IIb)—Medullary carcinoma of the thyroid, pheochromocytoma, and oral and intestinal ganglioneuromatosis (mucosal neuromas). TPN

All MEN syndromes are autosomal dominantly inherited.

MEN I = 3 "P" organs (pancreas, pituitary, and parathyroid).

Chromosomal translocations

t(9, 22), or the Philadelphia chromosome, is associated with CML.

t(8, 14) is associated with Burkitt's lymphoma.

t(14, 18) is associated with follicular lymphomas.

Zollinger–Ellison syndrome

Gastrin-secreting tumor that is usually located in the pancreas. Causes recurrent ulcers. May be associated with MEN syndrome type I.

Multiple myeloma

Monoclonal plasma cell cancer that arises in the marrow and produces large amounts of IgG (55%) or IgA (25%). Most common 1° tumor arising within bone in adults. Destructive bone lesions and consequent hypercalcemia. Renal insufficiency, ↑ susceptibility to infection, and anemia. Ig light chains in urine (Bence Jones protein). Associated with primary amyloidosis, M protein spike, and punched-out lytic bone lesions on x-ray.

Pathology

HIGH-YIELD FACTS

Tumors of the adrenal medulla

Pheochromocytoma is the most common tumor of the adrenal medulla in adults.
Neuroblastoma is the most common tumor of the adrenal medulla in children, but it can occur anywhere along the sympathetic chain.

Pheochromocytomas may be associated with neurofibromatosis, MEN type II and MEN type III.

Pheochromocytoma

Most of these neoplasms secrete a combination of norepinephrine and epinephrine, causing hypercatecholamine symptoms, including secondary hypertension. Urinary VMA levels and plasma catecholamines are elevated. Associated with MEN type IIa and type III. Have a dusky color on gross pathology. Treated with α antagonists, especially phenoxyben-zamine, a nonselective, **irreversible** α blocker.

Rule of 10s:
  10% malignant
  10% bilateral
  10% extraadrenal
  10% calcify
  10% kids
  10% familial
Also discussed 10-fold more often than actually seen!

Pancoast's tumor

Carcinoma that occurs in apex of lung and may affect inferior cervical ganglion, causing Horner's syndrome.

Carcinoid syndrome

Rare syndrome caused by carcinoid tumors, especially those of the small bowel; the tumors secrete high levels of serotonin that does not get metabolized by the liver due to liver metastases. Results in recurrent diarrhea, cutaneous flushing, asthmatic wheezing, and carcinoid heart disease.

Metastasis to bone

These primary tumors metastasize to bone: Breast, Lung, Thyroid, Testes, Kidney, Prostate.
Metastasis from breast and prostate are most common. Metastatic bone tumors are far more common than 1° bone tumors.

BLT[2] with a Kosher Pickle

Metastasis to brain

These primary tumors metastasize to brain: lung (bronchogenic carcinoma) > breast > skin (melanoma) > kidney (renal cell carcinoma) > GI tract. Overall, 25 to 30% of brain tumors are from metastases.

Metastasis to liver

The liver is the second most common site of metastasis after the regional lymph nodes. These primary tumors metastasize to the liver: colon (42%), stomach (23%), pancreas (21%), breast (14%), and lung (13%).

Metastatic liver tumors are far more common than primary liver tumors.

Hepatocellular carcinoma	Also called hepatoma. It is the most common primary tumor of the liver in adults. Increased incidence of hepatocellular carcinoma is associated with hepatitis B/C, Wilson's disease, hemochromatosis, α_1-antitrypsin deficiency, alcoholic cirrhosis, and carcinogens (e.g., aflatoxin B1).	Hepatocellular carcinoma, like renal cell carcinoma, is primarily spread by hematogenous dissemination.

Cancer epidemiology

	Male	**Female**	Deaths from lung cancer have plateaued in males, but deaths continue to increase in females.
Incidence	Prostate (32%)	Breast (32%)	
	Lung (16%)	Lung (13%)	
	Colon and rectum (12%)	Colon and rectum (13%)	
Mortality	Lung (33%)	Lung (23%)	
	Prostate (13%)	Breast (18%)	

Achalasia	Failure of relaxation of lower esophageal sphincter due to loss of innervation (Auerbach's plexus). Causes progressive dysphagia. Barium swallow shows dilated esophagus with an area of distal stenosis. Associated with an increased risk of esophageal carcinoma.	*A-chalasia* = absence of relaxation. 2° achalasia may arise from Chagas' disease.
Hirschsprung's disease	Congenital megacolon characterized by absence of parasympathetic ganglion cells (Auerbach's and Meissner's plexuses) on intestinal biopsy. Due to failure of neural crest cell migration. Symptoms: chronic constipation, manifests early in life. Dilated portion of the colon proximal to the aganglionic segment.	Think of a giant spring that **sprung** in the colon.
Whipple's disease	Multisystem, affects mainly small bowel. Can also affect skin, joints, CNS, heart, liver, spleen. Small intestine infiltrated by PAS-positive macrophages containing rod-shaped bacilli. Symptoms: diarrhea, weight loss, polyarthritis, and lymphadenopathy. Affects mostly white adult males. Caused by *Tropheryma whippelli* and treated with antibiotics.	Mr. Whipple has diarrhea and can't squeeze the Charmin (arthritis).
Crohn's disease	Inflammation is mainly in the terminal ileum and cecum but can be anywhere along GI tract. Segmental involvement (skip lesions); transmural involvement; cobblestone mucosa; bowel wall thickening ("string sign" on x-ray); lymphoid infiltrates; noncaseating granulomas; linear ulcers, fissures, fistulas.	Also called regional enteritis or ileitis. **Transmural** and **skip lesions** are key.

Ulcerative colitis	Begins in rectum and extends proximally. Continuous involvement; microabscesses (crypt abscesses) and ulcers; pseudopolyps (inflamed mucosal tags). Inflammatory cell infiltration confined to mucosa and submucosa, not transmural.	*Colitis* = colon inflammation. Key is continuous cephalad progression; not transmural. Associated with increased risk of carcinoma of the colon and toxic megacolon.
Cirrhosis	Diffuse fibrosis of liver, destroys normal architecture. Nodular regeneration. Micronodular: nodules < 3 mm, uniform size. Macronodular: nodules > 3 mm, varied size. Causes portal hypertension, varices, ascites, splenomegaly, jaundice, encephalopathy, and is associated with an increased risk of hepatocellular carcinoma.	*Cirrho* = tawny yellow (Greek). Micronodular cirrhosis is due to chronic insult (e.g., alcohol), whereas macronodular is usually due to an acute insult (e.g., postinfectious or drug-induced hepatitis).
Alcoholic hepatitis	Swollen and necrotic hepatocytes, neutrophil infiltration, Mallory bodies (hyaline), fatty change, and fibrosis around central vein. SGOT (AST) to SGPT (ALT) ratio is usually greater than 2.	
Wilson's disease	Due to failure of copper to enter circulation in the form of ceruloplasmin. Leads to copper accumulation, especially in liver, brain, iris. Cirrhosis (micronodular to macronodular), Mallory bodies in liver. Neuronal degeneration in basal ganglia (especially putamen). Associated with dementia, asterixis (flapping tremor), and an increased risk of hepatocellular carcinoma.	↓ serum ceruloplasmin. Kayser–Fleischer rings (copper deposits in iris).
Hemochromatosis	Increased iron deposition in many organs. Classic triad of micronodular pigment cirrhosis, "bronze" diabetes, skin pigmentation. Results in CHF and an increased risk of hepatocellular carcinoma.	Total body iron may reach 50 g, enough to set off the metal detectors at airports.

Hereditary hyperbilirubinemias

Crigler–Najjar syndrome, type I	Absent UDP-glucuronyl transferase. Presents early in life. Findings: jaundice, kernicterus (bile brain), ↑ unconjugated bilirubin. Treatment: plasmapheresis and phototherapy.	
Gilbert's syndrome	Mildly ↓ UDP-glucuronyl transferase. Asymptomatic, but unconjugated bilirubin is elevated without overt hemolysis.	Crigler-Najjar type I is a severe disease. Gilbert's may represent a milder form. Rotor's syndrome is similar, but less severe and does not cause black liver.
Dubin-Johnson syndrome	Conjugated hyperbilirubinemia due to defective liver excretion. Grossly black liver.	

Gallstones

Form when solubilizing bile acids and lecithin are overwhelmed by increased cholesterol and/or bilirubin.

Three types of stones:

1. Cholesterol stones: Associated with obesity, Crohn's disease, cystic fibrosis, advanced age, clofibrate, estrogens, multiparity, rapid weight loss and Native American origin.
2. Mixed stones: Have both cholesterol and pigment components.
3. Pigment stones: Seen in patients with chronic RBC hemolysis, cirrhosis, advanced age, and biliary infection.

Risk factors (5 Fs):
1. Female
2. Fat
3. Fertile
4. Forty
5. Flatulent

Degenerative diseases

Cerebral cortex	**Alzheimer's disease**—Most common cause of dementia in the elderly. Associated with senile plaques (β amyloid core) and neurofibrillary tangles (abnormally phosphorylated tau protein). Familial form (10%) associated with β-APP gene (chromosome 21) and Apo-E4 allele (chromosome 19).	Multi-infarct dementia is the second most common cause of dementia in the elderly.
	Pick's disease—Associated with Pick bodies and is specific for the frontal and temporal lobes.	
Basal ganglia and brainstem	**Huntington's disease**—Autosomal dominant inheritance, chorea, dementia.	
	Parkinson's disease—Associated with Lewy bodies and depigmentation of the substantia nigra. Can be caused by exposure to MPTP, a contaminant in illicit street drugs.	Parkinsonian symptoms (**RAFT**): Cogwheel **R**igidity, **A**kinesia, **F**lat facies, and **T**remor
Spinocerebellar	**Olivopontocerebellar atrophy**	
	Friedreich's ataxia	
Motor neuron	**Amyotrophic lateral sclerosis (ALS)**	ALS is associated with both lower and upper motor neuron signs.
	Werdnig-Hoffmann disease—Presents at birth as a "floppy baby"; tongue fasciculations.	
	Polio—Lower motor neuron signs.	

Demyelinating diseases

1. Multiple sclerosis—Higher prevalence in northern latitudes; periventricular plaques, preservation of axons, loss of oligodendrocytes, reactive astrocytic gliosis; ↑ protein (IgG) in CSF
2. Progressive multifocal leukoencephalopathy—Associated with JC virus and seen in 2–4% of AIDS
3. Postinfectious encephalomyelitis
4. Metachromatic leukodystrophy (a sphingolipidosis)
5. Guillain-Barré syndrome—Inflammation and demyelination of peripheral nerves; ascending muscle weakness and paralysis beginning in distal lower extremities

Wernicke-Korsakoff syndrome

Caused by vitamin B_1 deficiency in alcoholics. Classically may present with triad of psychosis, ophthalmoplegia, and ataxia (Wernicke's encephalopathy). May progress to memory loss, confabulation, confusion (Korsakoff's syndrome; irreversible). Associated with lesions in mamillary bodies.
Treatment: IV vitamin B_1 (thiamine).

Broca's versus Wernicke's aphasia

Broca's is nonfluent aphasia with intact comprehension (expressive aphasia). Wernicke's is fluent aphasia with impaired comprehension (receptive aphasia).

BROca's is **BRO**ken speech, Wernicke's is **W**ordy but makes no sense.

Horner's syndrome	Sympathectomy of face: 1. Ptosis (slight drooping of eyelid) 2. Miosis (pupil constriction) 3. Anhidrosis (absence of sweating) and flushing (rubor) of affected side of face Associated with Pancoast's tumor.
Arnold-Chiari deformity	Congenital protrusion of cerebellum and medulla through foramen magnum. Associated with meningomyelocele and obstructive hydrocephalus.

Syringomyelia	Softening and cavitation around central canal of spinal cord. Crossing fibers of spinothalamic tract are damaged. Bilateral loss of pain and temperature sensation in upper extremities with preservation of touch sensation.	*Syrinx* = tube (Greek) as in syringe.
Tabes dorsalis	Degeneration of dorsal columns and dorsal roots due to 3° syphilis, resulting in impaired proprioception and locomotor ataxia. Associated with Charcot's joints, shooting (lightning) pain, Argyll-Robertson pupils, and absence of deep tendon reflexes.	*Tabes* = wasting away (Latin).

PATHOLOGY—RHEUMATIC/AUTOIMMUNE

Osteoarthritis	Findings: destruction of articular cartilage (primarily weight-bearing joints), Heberden's nodes, eburnation, subchondral bone formation, sclerosis, osteophytes. Caused by wear and tear of joints. Classically hurts in evening after joint use.
Rheumatoid arthritis	Findings: pannus formation in joints (metacarpophalangeal, proximal interphalangeal); ulnar deviation, subluxation; subcutaneous rheumatoid nodules at pressure points (e.g., elbows); morning stiffness (decreased pain with use); symmetric involvement; positive rheumatoid factor (IgM). More common in females and is associated with HLA-DR4.
Gout	Precipitation of monosodium urate crystals into joints due to hyperuricemia. Asymmetric joint distribution. Favored site is big toe at the first MTP joint (podagra). Crystals are needle-shaped and negatively birefringent. Tophus formation. Hyperuricemia can be caused by Lesch-Nyhan disease, PRPP excess, decreased excretion of uric acid, or G6P deficiency. Treatment is colchicine and NSAIDs. Gout is associated with the use of thiazide diuretics, since they competitively inhibit the secretion of uric acid.

Systemic lupus erythematosus

90% are female. Fever, fatigue, weight loss. Joint pain, malar rash, pleuritis, pericarditis, nonbacterial verrucous endocarditis, Raynaud's phenomenon. **Wire loop** lesions in kidney with immune complex deposition (with nephrotic syndrome); death from renal failure and infections. Lab tests detect presence of:

1. Antinuclear antibodies (ANA): sensitive, but not specific for SLE
2. Antibodies to double-stranded DNA (anti-ds DNA): very specific
3. Anti-Smith antibodies (anti-Sm): very specific

Lupus = wolf (Latin), a reference to the malar rash (on cheeks) causing wolf-like facies. Also, **wire loopus** erythematosus.

Sarcoidosis

Associated with restrictive lung disease, bilateral hilar lymphadenopathy, erythema nodosum, Bell's palsy, epithelial granulomas containing microscopic Schaumann and asteroid bodies, uveoparotitis, and hypercalcemia (due to elevated conversion of vit. D_3 to its active form in epithelioid macrophages). Also associated with immune-mediated widespread noncaseating granulomas and elevated serum ACE levels.

Sarko = flesh (Greek), describing exuberant noncaseating granulomas. Common in black females.

Scleroderma (progressive systemic sclerosis-PSS)

Excessive fibrosis throughout the body. 75% female. Commonly sclerosis of skin, but also of cardiovascular and GI systems, kidney. Two major categories:

1. Diffuse scleroderma: widespread skin involvement, rapid progression, early visceral involvement. Associated with ANA anti-Scl-70.
2. **CREST** syndrome: **C**alcinosis, **R**aynaud's phenomenon, **E**sophageal dysmotility, **S**clerodactyly, and **T**elangiectasia. Limited skin involvement, often confined to fingers and face. More benign clinical course. Associated with anticentromere antibody.

Goodpasture's syndrome

Findings: pulmonary hemorrhages, renal lesions, hemoptysis, hematuria, anemia, proliferative glomerulonephritis, crescents.
Anti-glomerular basement membrane antibodies produce linear staining on immunofluorescence.

There are two good pastures for this disease: glomerulus and pulmonary. Also, a type II hypersensitivity disease. Mostly affects men in 20s and 30s.

Reiter's syndrome

A seronegative spondyloarthropathy. Strong HLA-B27 link. Classic triad:

1. Urethritis
2. Conjunctivitis and anterior uveitis
3. Arthritis

Has a strong predilection for males.

"Can't see (anterior uveitis/ conjunctivitis), can't pee (urethritis), can't climb a tree (arthritis)."

Sjögren's syndrome	Classic triad: dry eyes (conjunctivitis, xerophthalmia), dry mouth (dysphagia, xerostomia), arthritis. Parotid enlargement, ↑ risk of B-cell lymphoma. Predominantly affects females between 40 and 60 years of age.	Associated with rheumatoid arthritis.
Reye's syndrome	Rare, often fatal childhood encephalopathy. Findings: fatty liver (microvesicular fatty change), hypoglycemia, coma. Associated with viral infection (especially VZV and influenza B) and salicylates; thus aspirin is no longer recommended for children and acetaminophen is given instead.	Encephalopathy and liver failure

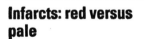

PATHOLOGY—VASCULAR/CARDIAC

Intracranial hemorrhage

Epidural hematoma	Rupture of middle meningeal artery, often 2° to fracture of temporal bone.
Subdural hematoma	Rupture of bridging veins. Venous bleeding (less pressure) with delayed onset of symptoms. Seen in elderly individuals, alcoholics, blunt trauma.
Subarachnoid hemorrhage	Rupture of an aneurysm (usually berry aneurysm) or an AVM. Patients complain of "worst headache ever." Bloody or xanthochromic spinal tap.
Parenchymal hematoma	Caused by HTN, amyloid angiopathy and tumor.

Berry aneurysms	Berry aneurysms occur at the bifurcations in the circle of Willis. Most common site is bifurcation of the anterior communicating artery. Rupture (most common complication) leads to hemorrhagic stroke. Associated with adult polycystic kidney.	Red berries at bifurcations bulge and blow out.
Infarcts: red versus pale	Red (hemorrhagic) infarcts occur in loose tissues with collaterals, such as lungs, intestine, and brain, or following reperfusion. Pale infarcts occur in solid tissues with single blood supply, such as heart, kidney, and spleen.	REd = REperfusion.

Evolution of MI

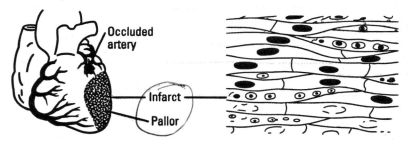

Coronary artery occlusion: LAD > RCA > circumflex

A. First day

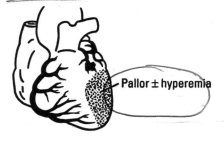

Occluded artery

Infarct

Pallor

Coagulative necrosis leads to release of contents of necrotic cells into bloodstream

Muscle shows minimal changes

B. 2 to 4 days

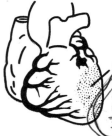

Pallor ± hyperemia

Tissue surrounding infarct shows acute inflammation

Dilated vessels (hyperemia)

Neutrophil emigration

Muscle shows microscopic changes of coagulative necrosis

C. 5 to 10 days

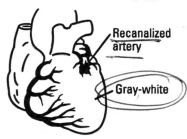

Hyperemic border; central yellow-brown softening— maximally yellow and soft by 10 days

Outer zone (ingrowth of granulation tissue)

Macrophage zone

Neutrophil zone

D. 7 weeks

Recanalized artery

Gray-white

Contracted scar complete

MI lab values

CK-MB is test of choice in the first 24 hours post-MI.
LDH$_1$ is test of choice from 2 to 7 days post-MI.
AST is nonspecific and can be found in cardiac, liver, and skeletal muscle cells.

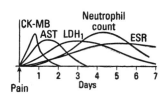

MI complications

1. Cardiac arrhythmia (90%)
2. LV failure and pulmonary edema (60%)
3. Thromboembolism: mural thrombus
4. Cardiogenic shock
5. Rupture of ventricular free wall, interventricular septum, papillary muscle (4–7 days post-MI)
6. Fibrinous pericarditis: friction rub (3–5 days post-MI)
7. Dressler's syndrome: autoimmune phenomenon resulting in fibrinous pericarditis (several weeks post-MI)

CHF

Abnormality	Cause
Ankle, sacral edema	RV failure → increased venous pressure → fluid transudation.
Hepatomegaly	Increased venous pressure → increased resistance to portal flow.
Pulmonary congestion	LV failure → increased pulmonary venous pressure → pulmonary venous distention and transudation of fluid.
Dyspnea on exertion	Failure of left ventricular output to increase during exercise.
Paroxysmal dyspnea, pulmonary edema	Failure of left heart output to keep up with right heart output → acute rise in pulmonary venous and capillary pressure → transudation of fluid.
Orthopnea	Pooling of blood in lungs in supine position adds volume to congested pulmonary vascular system; increased venous return not put out by left ventricle.
Cardiac dilation	Greater ventricular end-diastolic volume.

Decreased myocardial contractility
↓
Decreased cardiac output
↓
↓ Effective arterial blood volume
↙ ↘
↑ Sympathetic nervous outflow → ↑ Renin release
→ Maintains blood pressure ← Angiotensin II
↑ Venous pressure → Renal vasoconstriction ← ↑ Aldosterone secretion
↓ GFR → ↑ Tubular reabsorption of Na⁺ and H₂O
↓ Urinary excretion of Na⁺ and H₂O
↑ Total body Na⁺ and H₂O
Edema

Embolus types

Fat, **A**ir, **T**hrombus, **B**acteria, **A**mniotic fluid, **T**umor. Fat emboli are associated with long bone fractures. Amniotic fluid emboli can lead to DIC, especially postpartum.

An embolus moves like a **FAT BAT.** Approximately 95% of pulmonary emboli arise from deep leg veins.

Bacterial endocarditis	New murmur, anemia, fever, Osler nodes. Multiple blood cultures necessary for diagnosis (continuous bacteremia). 1. Acute: *Staphylococcus aureus* (high virulence). Large vegetations on previously normal valves. 2. Subacute: *Streptococcus viridans* (low virulence). Smaller vegetations on congenitally abnormal or diseased valves.	Mitral valve is most frequently involved. Tricuspid valve endocarditis is associated with IV drug abuse.
Marantic endocarditis (nonbacterial)	Fibrin precipitation on valve leaflets, 2° to metastasis, renal failure, or sepsis. Vegetations are small and sterile but can produce emboli and infarctions.	
Rheumatic fever/ rheumatic heart disease	Rheumatic fever is a consequence of pharyngeal infection with group A, β-hemolytic streptococci. Multiple episodes can cause rheumatic heart disease, which affects heart valves: mitral > aortic >> tricuspid. Associated with Aschoff bodies, migratory polyarthritis, erythema marginatum, elevated ASO titers.	**PH**ever follows **PH**aryngeal infection. High-pressure valves are affected most.
Pericarditis	Causes: infection (viruses, TB, pyogenic bacteria, often by direct spread from lung or mediastinal lymph nodes), ischemic heart disease, chronic renal failure → uremia, and connective tissue disease. Effusions are usually serous; hemorrhagic effusions are associated with renal failure, TB, and malignancy. Findings: pericardial pain, friction rub. Can resolve without scarring or lead to chronic adhesive or chronic constrictive pericarditis.	
Pancytopenia	Pancytopenia is associated with the following pathologic conditions: 1. AML 2. Recurrent ovarian cancer 3. Aplastic anemia	
Diagnosis of congenital hematologic defects	Heinz bodies are seen in G6PD deficiency. Ham's test is used to diagnose paroxysmal nocturnal hemoglobinuria (PNH). Osmotic fragility test is used to diagnose hereditary spherocytosis.	

Pathology

HIGH-YIELD FACTS

Ischemic heart disease	Possible manifestations: 1. Angina: Stable: mostly 2° to atherosclerosis 　　　Prinzmetal's variant: occurs at rest, 2° to coronary artery spasm 　　　Unstable/crescendo: thrombosis in a branch 2. Myocardial infarction—most often occurs in CAD involving the left anterior descending artery 3. Sudden cardiac death—death from cardiac causes within 1 hour of onset of symptoms, most commonly due to a lethal arrhythmia 4. Chronic ischemic heart disease—progressive onset of congestive heart failure over many years due to chronic ischemic myocardial damage	
Atherosclerosis	Disease of elastic arteries and large and medium-sized muscular arteries. Risk factors: smoking, hypertension, diabetes mellitus, hyperlipidemia, obesity Progression: fatty streaks → doxorubicin → complex atheromas. Complications: aneurysms, ischemia, infarcts, peripheral vascular disease, thrombus, emboli. Location: abdominal aorta > coronary artery > popliteal artery > carotid artery Symptoms: angina, claudication, but can be asymptomatic.	
Cardiomyopathies		
Dilated (congestive) cardiomyopathy	Most common cardiomyopathy (90% of cases). Etiologies include EtOH toxicity, postviral myocarditis by coxsackievirus B, doxorubicin toxicity, beriberi, peripartum cardiomyopathy, chronic cocaine use. Heart dilates and looks like a balloon on chest x-ray.	Systolic dysfunction ensues.
Hypertrophic cardiomyopathy	Hypertrophy often asymmetric and involving the intraventricular septum. 50% of cases are familial and are inherited as an AD trait. Walls of LV are thickened and chamber becomes banana-shaped on x-ray.	Also referred to as IHSS, or idiopathic hypertrophic subaortic stenosis. Diastolic dysfunction ensues.
Restrictive/obliterative cardiomyopathy	Major causes include sarcoidosis, amyloidosis, endocardial fibroelastosis, and endomyocardial fibrosis (Löffler's).	
Syphilitic heart disease	Tertiary syphilis disrupts the vasa vasorum of aorta via endarteritis obliterans and disrupts elastica (with consequent dilation of aorta and valve ring). Often affects the aortic root and ascending aorta. Associated with a tree-bark appearance of the aorta.	Can result in aneurysm of ascending aorta or aortic arch and aortic valve incompetence.
Buerger's disease	Known as smoker's disease and thromboangiitis obliterans: idiopathic, segmental, thrombosing vasculitis of intermediate and small peripheral arteries and veins. Findings: intermittent claudication, superficial nodular phlebitis, cold sensitivity (Raynaud's phenomenon), severe pain in affected part; may lead to gangrene. Treatment: quit smoking.	

Takayasu's arteritis — Known as "pulseless disease": thickening of aortic arch and/or proximal great vessels, causing weak pulses in upper extremities and ocular disturbances. Associated with an elevated ESR. Primarily affects young Asian females. — Affects medium and large arteries.

Temporal arteritis — Most common vasculitis which affects medium and small arteries, usually branches of carotid artery. Findings include jaw claudication and possible occlusion of ophthalmic artery, leading to blindness. Half of patients have systemic involvement and syndrome of polymyalgia rheumatica. Associated with unilateral headaches and elevated ESR. — Temporal = signs near **temples**. ESR is markedly elevated. Also known as giant cell arteritis.

Budd-Chiari syndrome — Occlusion of IVC or hepatic veins with centrilobular congestion and necrosis, leading to congestive liver disease (hepatomegaly, ascites, abdominal pain, and eventual liver failure). Associated with polycythemia vera, pregnancy, hepatocellular carcinoma.

PATHOLOGY—OTHER

Glomerular pathology

Nephritic syndrome: Hematuria, hypertension, oliguria.
1. Acute poststreptococcal glomerulonephritis—
   LM: glomeruli enlarged and hypercellular; neutrophils.
   EM: subepithelial humps. IF: granular pattern. — Most frequently seen in children.
2. Rapidly progressive (crescentic) glomerulonephritis—
   LM and IF: "crescent moon" shape.
3. Goodpasture's syndrome—IF: linear pattern.
4. Membranoproliferative glomerulonephritis—
   EM: subendothelial humps.
5. IgA nephropathy (Berger's disease)—IF and EM:
   mesangial deposits of IgA.

Nephrotic syndrome: Massive proteinuria, hypoalbuminemia, generalized edema, hyperlipidemia
1. Membranous glomerulonephritis—LM: diffuse capillary thickening. IF: granular pattern. — Most common cause of adult nephrotic syndrome.
2. Minimal change disease (lipoid nephrosis)— LM: normal glomeruli. EM: foot process effacement (fusion). — Most common cause of childhood nephrotic syndrome.
3. Focal segmental glomerulonephritis—LM: segmental sclerosis and hyalinosis.

(**LM** = light microscopy; **EM** = electron microscopy; **IF** = immunofluorescence)

Cretinism	Endemic cretinism occurs wherever endemic goiter is prevalent (lack of dietary iodine); sporadic cretinism is caused by defect in T4 formation or developmental failure in thyroid formation. Findings: pot-bellied, pale, puffy-faced child with protruding umbilicus and protuberant tongue.	Cretin means Christ-like (French *chretien*). Those affected were considered so mentally retarded as to be incapable of sinning.
Hydatidiform mole	A pathologic ovum ("empty egg"—ovum with no DNA) resulting in cystic swelling of chorionic villi and proliferation of chorionic epithelium (trophoblast). Most common precursor of choriocarcinoma. High β-HCG. "Honeycombed uterus," "cluster of grapes" appearance. Genotype of a complete mole is 46,XX and is purely paternal in origin (no maternal chromosomes).	
Asbestosis	Diffuse pulmonary interstitial fibrosis caused by inhaled asbestos fibers. Increased risk of pleural mesothelioma and bronchogenic carcinoma. Long latency. Ferruginous bodies in lung (asbestos fibers coated with hemosiderin). Ivory-white pleural plaques.	Smokers have synergistically higher risk of cancer.
Neonatal respiratory distress syndrome	Surfactant deficiency leading to ↑ surface tension resulting in alveolar collapse. Surfactant is made by type II cells most abundantly after 35th wk gestation. The lecithin to sphingomyelin ratio in the amniotic fluid, a measure of lung maturity, is usually less than 1.5 in neonatal respiratory distress syndrome.	

PATHOLOGY—FINDINGS

Aortic insufficiency	Pistol shot sound heard over femoral vessels (Traube sign). Water hammer pulse over carotid artery (Corrigan pulse). Quincke's capillary pulsations (pressure on fingernail results in visible pulsations).	
Argyll-Robertson pupil	Argyll-Robertson pupil constricts with accommodation but not reactive to light. Pathognomonic for 3° syphilis.	**Argyll-Robertson Pupil** **ARP: A**ccommodation **R**esponse **P**resent **PRA: P**upillary (light) **R**eflex **A**bsent
Aschoff body	Aschoff bodies (granuloma with giant cells) and Anitschkow's cells (histiocytes around the granuloma) are found in rheumatic heart disease.	Think of two **RH**ussians with **RH**eumatic heart disease (Aschoff and Anitschkow).
Auer bodies (rods)	Auer rods are cytoplasmic inclusions in granulocytes and myeloblasts. Primarily seen in acute promyelocytic leukemia. *AML*	

Casts	Casts of nephron: RBC casts = glomerular inflammation, ischemia, or malignant hypertension. WBC casts = inflammation in renal interstitium, tubules, and glomeruli. Hyaline casts often seen in normal urine.	RBC = glomeruli.
Erythrocyte sedimentation rate	Very nonspecific test that measures acute phase reactants. Dramatically increased with infection, malignancy, connective tissue disease. Also increased with pregnancy, inflammatory disease, anemia. Decreased with sickle cell anemia, polycythemia, congestive heart failure.	Simple, cheap, but nonspecific. Should not be used for asymptomatic screening; can be used to diagnose and monitor temporal arteritis and polymyalgia rheumatica.
Ghon complex	TB granulomas with lobar or perihilar lymph node involvement (Ghon focus and lymph node involvement). Reflects primary infection or exposure.	Ghon complex is the lung and the node; Ghon focus is just the focus of lung involvement.
Hyperlipidemia signs	Atheromata = plaques in blood vessel walls. Xanthelasma = Plaques or nodules composed of lipid-laden histiocytes in the skin, especially the eyelids. Tendinous xanthoma = lipid deposit in tendon, especially Achilles. Corneal arcus = lipid deposit in cornea, nonspecific (arcus senilis).	
Psammoma bodies	Laminated, concentric, calcific spherules seen in: 1. Papillary adenocarcinoma of thyroid 2. Serous papillary cystadenocarcinoma of ovary 3. Meningioma 4. Malignant mesothelioma	**P**apillary (thyroid) **S**erous (ovary) **a** **M**eningioma **M**esothelioma
RBC forms	Biconcave = normal. Spherocytes = hereditary spherocytosis, autoimmune hemolysis. Elliptocyte = hereditary elliptocytosis. Macro-ovalocyte = megaloblastic anemia, marrow failure. Helmet cell, schistocyte = DIC, traumatic hemolysis. Sickle cell = sickle cell anemia.	
Target cell	Most commonly indicates hemolytic anemia, thalassemia, hemoglobinopathies, sickle cell anemia, or liver disease.	Looks like a shooting target (bull's-eye).
Roth's spots	White spots of coagulated fibrin in retina seen on fundoscopic exam. Associated with bacterial endocarditis.	

Sentinel loop (x-ray)	Represents a distended bowel loop suggestive of a localized ileus secondary to an inflamed abdominal viscus, as in pancreatitis, appendicitis, cholecystitis.
Virchow's (sentinel) node	A firm supraclavicular lymph node, often on left side, easily palpable (can be detected by medical students), also known as "jugular gland." Presumptive evidence of malignant visceral neoplasm (classically stomach).

Anemia

Type	Etiology	
Microcytic, hypochromic	Iron deficiency: ↑ transferrin, ↓ ferritin, ↓ serum iron Anemia of chronic disease: ↓ transferrin, ↑ ferritin, ↓ serum iron, ↑ storage iron in marrow macrophages. Thalassemias Lead poisoning	Vit. B_{12} and folate deficiencies are associated with hypersegmented PMNs. Unlike folate deficiency, vit. B_{12} deficiency is associated with neurological problems.
Macrocytic	Megaloblastic: Vitamin B_{12}/folate deficiency Drugs that block DNA synthesis (eg, sulfa drugs, AZT) Marked reticulocytosis	Serum haptoglobin and serum LDH are used to determine RBC hemolysis. Direct Coombs' test is used to distinguish between immune vs. nonimmune mediated RBC hemolysis.
Normocytic, normochromic	Hemorrhage Enzyme defects (eg, G6PD deficiency, PK deficiency) RBC membrane defects (eg, hereditary spherocytosis) Bone marrow disorders (eg, aplastic anemia, leukemia) Hemoglobinopathies (eg, sickle cell disease) Autoimmune hemolytic anemia	

Congenital
1. Maternal complications of birth (e.g., Sheehan's syndrome, puerperal infection).
2. Clinical manifestations and complications of cystic fibrosis.

Neoplastic
1. Hormone-producing neoplasms (e.g., small cell carcinoma of the lung, carcinoid).
2. Common malignant skin diseases (e.g., basal cell carcinoma, melanoma, squamous cell carcinoma).
3. Leading bone tumors (e.g., metastasis, giant cell tumor).
4. Clinical manifestations of lymphomas (e.g., Burkitt's and non-Hodgkin's lymphomas).
5. Risk factors for common carcinomas (e.g., lung, breast).
6. Carcinogenic chemicals (e.g., vinyl chloride, nitrosamines, aflatoxin B1).
7. Malignancies associated with pulmonary pneumoconiosis (e.g., asbestosis, silicosis).
8. AIDS-associated neoplasms (Kaposi's sarcoma, non-Hodgkin's lymphoma).

Nervous
1. Types of hydrocephalus (e.g., communicating).
2. CNS manifestations of viral infections such as HSV and HIV.
3. Spinal muscular atrophies (e.g., Werdnig-Hoffman disease, Lou Gehrig's disease).

Rheumatic/Autoimmune
1. Rheumatic fever.
2. Transplant rejection (e.g., hyperacute reactions, graft-versus-host disease).
3. Differences between rheumatoid arthritis and degenerative joint disease.

Vascular/Hematology
1. Complications of hypertension (e.g., cerebral vascular accidents, renal disease).
2. Common hematologic diseases (e.g., thrombocytopenia, clotting factor deficiencies, lymphoma, and leukemia).
3. Different types of vasculitis (e.g., Kawasaki disease, Wegener's granulomatosis, polyarteritis nodosa, hypersensitivity angiitis).
4. Heart valve diseases (e.g., mitral stenosis, aortic insufficiency, patent ductus arteriosus), including associated murmurs.
5. Pathophysiology of thoracic versus abdominal aortic aneurysm.

General
1. Common clinical features of AIDS (e.g., central nervous system, pulmonary, gastrointestinal, dermatologic).
2. Adult and infant respiratory distress syndromes.

3. Mechanism and consequences of vesicoureteral reflux.
4. Types of necrosis and the common organs involved (e.g., coagulation necrosis, liquefactive necrosis).
5. Esophageal reflux disease.
6. Differences between duodenal and gastric ulcers.
7. Causes and risk factors for intestinal obstruction (e.g., intussusception, volvulus, imperforated anus).
8. Clinical symptoms and laboratory findings of gout and pseudogout.
9. Risk factors of pulmonary embolism.
10. Differences between Cushing's syndrome and Cushing's disease.
11. Common sequelae of diabetes mellitus, types I and II.
12. Chemical mediators of inflammation (e.g., histamine, prostaglandins, kinin system).
13. Common sequelae of smoking.

Pharmacology

Preparation for questions on pharmacology is straightforward. Memorizing all the key drugs and their characteristics (e.g., mechanisms, clinical use) is high yield. Focus on understanding the prototype drugs in each class. Avoid memorizing obscure derivatives. Learn the "classic" and distinguishing toxicities of the major drugs. Do not bother with drug dosages or trade names. There is a strong emphasis on autonomic nervous system, central nervous system, antimicrobial, and cardiovascular agents. Much of the material is clinically relevant.

Antimicrobial
CNS
Cardiovascular
Cancer Drugs
Toxicology
Miscellaneous
High-Yield Topics

Penicillin

Penicillin G (IV form), penicillin V (oral)

Mechanism
1. Binds penicillin-binding proteins
2. Blocks transpeptidase cross-linking of cell wall
3. Activates autolytic enzymes

Clinical use
Bactericidal for gram-positive cocci, gram-positive rods, gram-negative cocci, and spirochetes. Not penicillinase resistant.

Toxicity
Hypersensitivity reactions.

Methicillin, nafcillin, dicloxacillin

Mechanism
Same as penicillin. Narrow spectrum, penicillinase resistant because of bulkier R group.

Clinical use
Staphylococcus aureus.

Toxicity
Hypersensitivity reactions; methicillin: interstitial nephritis.

Ampicillin, amoxicillin

Mechanism
Same as penicillin. Wider spectrum, penicillinase sensitive. Also, combine with clavulanic acid (penicillinase inhibitor) to enhance spectrum. Amoxicillin has a greater oral bioavailability than ampicillin.

Coverage: ampicillin/amoxicillin **"HELPS"**

Clinical use
Extended-spectrum penicillin: Certain gram-positive bacteria and gram-negative rods (*Haemophilus influenzae*, *Escherichia coli*, *Listeria monocytogenes*, *Proteus mirabilis*, *Salmonella*).

Toxicity
Hypersensitivity reactions; ampicillin: rash.

Carbenicillin, ticarcillin

Mechanism
Same as penicillin. Extended spectrum.

Clinical use
Pseudomonas species and gram-negative rods.

Toxicity
Hypersensitivity reactions.

Cephalosporins

Mechanism
β-lactam drugs that inhibit cell wall synthesis but are less susceptible to penicillinases. Bactericidal.

1st generation: **PEcK**
2nd generation: **HEN PEcKS**

Clinical use
First generation: gram-positive cocci, *Proteus mirabilis*, *E. coli*, *Klebsiella pneumoniae*.

Second generation: gram-positive cocci, *Haemophilus influenzae*, *Enterobacter aerogenes*, *Neisseria* species, *Proteus mirabilis*, *E. coli*, *K. pneumoniae*, *Serratia marcescens*.

Third generation: Serious gram-negative infections. These drugs can penetrate into CNS.

Toxicity
Hypersensitivity reactions, increased nephrotoxicity of aminoglycosides, disulfiram-like reaction with ethanol (in cephalosporins with a methylthiotetrazole group).

Aztreonam

Mechanism	A monobactam resistant to β-lactamases. Inhibits cell wall synthesis (binds to PBP3). Synergistic with aminoglycosides. No cross-allergenicity with penicillins.
Clinical use	Gram-negative rods: *Klebsiella* species, *Pseudomonas* species, *Serratia* species. No activity against gram-positives or anaerobes.
Toxicity	GI upset with possible superinfections, vertigo, headache.

Imipenem

Mechanism	A carbapenem. Wide spectrum. β-lactamase resistant. Always administered with cilastatin (inhibitor of renal dihydropeptidase I).
Clinical use	Gram-positive cocci, gram-negative rods, and anaerobes.
Toxicity	GI distress, skin rash, and CNS toxicity (at high plasma levels).

Vancomycin

Mechanism	Inhibits cell wall mucopeptide formation. Bactericidal.
Clinical use	Used for serious, gram-positive multidrug-resistant organisms, including *Staphylococcus aureus* and *Clostridium difficile* (pseudomembranous colitis).
Toxicity	Nephrotoxicity, Ototoxicity, Thrombophlebitis, diffuse flushing—"red man syndrome" (can largely prevent by pretreatment with antihistamines and slow infusion rate). Well tolerated in general. Does **NOT** have many problems.

Protein synthesis inhibitors

"Buy **AT 30, CELL** at 50"

30S Inhibitors:

A = Aminoglycosides (streptomycin, gentamicin, tobramycin, amikacin) [bactericidal]

T = Tetracyclines [bacteriostatic]

50S Inhibitors:

C = Chloramphenicol [bacteriostatic]

E = Erythromycin [bacteriostatic]

L = Lincomycin [bacteriostatic]

L = cLindamycin [bacteriostatic]

Aminoglycosides

Gentamicin, streptomycin, tobramycin, amikacin

Mechanism	Bactericidal, inhibits formation of initiation complex and causes misreading of mRNA. Requires O_2 for uptake, therefore ineffective against anaerobes.
Clinical use	Severe gram-negative rod infections.
Toxicity	Ototoxicity (especially when used with loop diuretics), nephrotoxicity (especially when used with cephalosporins).

Tetracyclines

Tetracycline, doxycycline, demeclocycline, minocycline

Mechanism Bacteriostatic, binds to 30S and prevents attachment of aminoacyl-tRNA, limited CNS penetration. Doxycycline fecally eliminated and can be used in patients with renal failure. Must NOT take with milk or antacids because divalent cations inhibit its absorption in the gut.

Clinical use *Borrelia burgdorferi* (Lyme disease), *Chlamydia*, *Ureaplasma*, *Mycoplasma pneumoniae*, *Rickettsiae*, Acne, Tularemia, Cholera (*Vibrio cholerae*)

Coverage: **B CUM RATC**: "Become rats."

Toxicity GI distress, discolors teeth in children, inhibits bone growth in children, Fanconi's syndrome, photosensitivity.

Erythromycin

Mechanism Inhibits protein synthesis by blocking translocation, binds to the 23S rRNA of the 50S ribosomal subunit.
Bacteriostatic.

Clinical use Gram-positive cocci, *Mycoplasma*, *Legionella*, *Chlamydia*, *Neisseria*.

Toxicity Acute cholestatic hepatitis, eosinophilia, skin rashes.

Chloramphenicol

Mechanism Inhibits 50S peptidyl transferase. Bacteriostatic.

Clinical use Meningitis (*H. influenzae*, *Neisseria meningitidis*, *Streptococcus pneumoniae*).

Toxicity Anemia, aplastic anemia, gray baby syndrome (overdose in premature infants lacking liver UDP-glucuronyl transferase).

Sulfonamides

Sulfamethoxazole (SMZ), sulfisoxazole, triple sulfas

Mechanism PABA antimetabolites inhibit dihydropteroate synthetase. Bacteriostatic.

Clinical use Gram-positive, gram-negative, *Nocardia*, *Chlamydia*. Triple sulfas or SMZ for simple UTI.

Toxicity Hypersensitivity reactions, hemolysis if G6PD deficient, nephrotoxicity, kernicterus in infants, displace other drugs from albumin.

Trimethoprim

Mechanism Inhibits dihydrofolate reductase. Bacteriostatic.

Clinical use Used in combination with sulfonamides (trimethoprim-sulfamethoxazole), causing sequential block of folate synthesis. Combination used for recurrent UTI, *Shigella*, *Salmonella*, *Pneumocystis carinii* pneumonia.

Trimethoprim = **TMP**: "Treats Marrow Poorly."

Toxicity Megaloblastic anemia, leukopenia, granulocytopenia.

Fluoroquinolones

 Ciprofloxacin and norfloxacin (fluoroquinolones), nalidixic acid (a quinolone).

Mechanism Inhibits DNA gyrase (topoisomerase II). Bactericidal.

Clinical use Gram-negative rods (including *Pseudomonas*), *Neisseria*, some gram-positive organisms.

Toxicity GI upset, superinfections, skin rashes, headache, dizziness. Contraindicated in pregnancy and children because of damage to cartilage.

Metronidazole
Mechanism	Forms toxic metabolites in the bacterial cell. Bactericidal.
Clinical use	Antiprotozoal, trichomoniasis, giardiasis, amebiasis, *Gardnerella vaginalis*, anaerobes (*Bacteroides, Clostridium*). Used with bismuth and amoxicillin or tetracycline for "triple therapy" against *H. pylori*.
Toxicity	Disulfiram-like reaction with alcohol, vestibular dysfunction, headache.

Polymyxins
Polymyxin B, polymyxin E
Mechanism	Bind to cell membranes of bacteria and disrupt their osmotic properties. Polymyxins are cationic, basic proteins that act like detergents.
Clinical use	Resistant gram-negative cocci, gram-negative rods.
Toxicity	Neurotoxicity, acute renal tubular necrosis.

Isoniazid (INH)
Mechanism	Decreases synthesis of mycolic acids.	**INH:**
Clinical use	*Mycobacterium tuberculosis*. The only agent used as solo prophylaxis against TB.	Injures **N**eurons and **H**epatocytes.
Toxicity	Hemolysis if G6PD deficient, neurotoxicity, hepatotoxicity. Pyridoxine (vit. B$_6$) can prevent neurotoxicity.	

Rifampin
Mechanism	Inhibits DNA-dependent RNA polymerase.	**Rifampin's 4 R's:**
Clinical use	*M. tuberculosis*, delays resistance to dapsone when used for leprosy. Always used in combination with other drugs except in the treatment of meningococcal carrier state, and chemoprophylaxis in contacts of children with *H. influenzae* type B.	**R**NA polymerase inhibitor **R**evs up microsomal P450 **R**ed/orange body fluids **R**apid resistance if used alone
Toxicity	Increased elimination of anticoagulants and methadone, hepatotoxicity, thrombocytopenia, skin rashes, flu response, decreased antibody responses.	

Amphotericin B
Mechanism	Binds ergosterol (unique to fungi), forms membrane pores that disrupt homeostasis.
Clinical use	*Cryptococcus, Blastomyces, Coccidioides, Histoplasma, Candida, Mucor* (systemic mycoses). Intrathecally for fungal meningitis; does not cross blood–brain barrier.
Toxicity	Fever, chills, hypotension, nephrotoxicity, arrhythmias ("amphoterrible").

Fluconazole, ketoconazole, clotrimazole, miconazole
Mechanism	Inhibits fungal steroid synthesis.
Clinical use	Fluconazole for cryptococcus in AIDS patients and candidal infections of all types. Ketoconazole for *Blastomyces, Coccidioides, Histoplasma, C. albicans*.
Toxicity	Hormone synthesis inhibition (gynecomastia), liver dysfunction (inhibits cyt. P450), fever, chills.

Griseofulvin

Mechanism	Interference with microtubule function, disrupts mitosis. Deposits in keratin-containing tissues (e.g., nails).
Clinical use	Oral treatment of superficial infections, inhibits growth of dermatophytes and *C. albicans.*
Toxicity	Teratogenic, carcinogenic, confusion, headaches, ↑ coumarin metabolism.

Amantadine

Mechanism	Blocks viral penetration/uncoating; may buffer pH of endosome. Also causes the release of dopamine from intact nerve terminals.	**A**mantadine blocks influenza **A** and *Rubell***A** and causes problems with the cerebell**A.**
Clinical use	Prophylaxis for influenza A and rubella. Parkinson's disease.	
Toxicity	Ataxia, dizziness, slurred speech.	

Acyclovir

Mechanism	Preferentially inhibits viral DNA polymerase when phosphorylated by viral thymidine kinase.
Clinical use	HSV, VZV, EBV. Mucocutaneous and genital herpes lesions. Prophylaxis in immunocompromised patients.
Toxicity	Delirium, tremor, renal crystals.

Ganciclovir

DHPG (dihydroxy-2-propoxymethyl guanine)

Mechanism	Phosphorylation by viral kinase preferentially inhibits CMV DNA polymerase.
Clinical use	CMV, especially in immunocompromised patients.
Toxicity	Leukopenia, thrombocytopenia, renal toxicity.

Zidovudine (AZT)

Mechanism	Preferentially inhibits reverse transcriptase of HIV.	**AZT: A**lways **Z**aps
Clinical use	HIV-infected patients.	**T**hrombocytes.
Toxicity	Thrombocytopenia, granulocytopenia, anemia.	

Antiparasitic drugs

Ivermectin	Onchocerciasis ("river blindness" ⇒ r**IVER**-mectin).
Mebendazole	Nematode/roundworm (e.g., pinworm and whipworm) infections.
Praziquantel	Trematode/fluke (e.g., schistosomes, *Paragonimus, Clonorchis,* cysticerci) infections.
Niclosamide	Cestode/tapeworm (e.g., *D. latum, Taenia* species) infections.
Pentavalent antimony	Leishmaniasis.
Chloroquine, quinine, mefloquine	Malaria.
Metronidazole	Giardiasis, amoebic dysentery (*E. histolytica*), bacterial vaginitis (*Gardnerella vaginalis*).
Pentamidine	*Pneumocystis carinii* pneumonia.
Nifurtimox	Chagas' disease (*Trypanosoma cruzi*).

Autonomic drugs

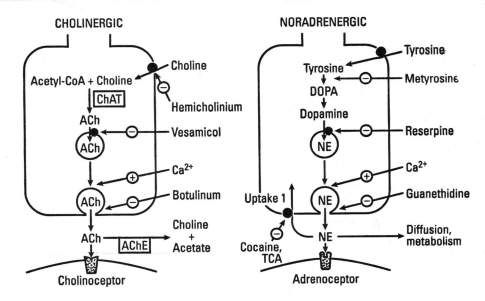

Solid circles represent transporters; ChAT, choline acetate transferase; ACh, acetylcholine; AChE, acetylcholinesterase; NE, norepinephrine.

Cholinomimetics

	Clinical Applications	Action
Direct agonists		
Bethanechol	Postoperative and neurogenic ileus and urinary retention	Activates bowel and bladder smooth muscle
Carbachol, pilocarpine	Glaucoma	Activates ciliary muscle of eye (open angle), pupillary sphincter (narrow angle)
Indirect agonists (anti-cholinesterases)		
Neostigmine	Postoperative and neurogenic ileus and urinary retention	↑ endogenous ACh
Neostigmine, pyridostigmine, edrophonium	Myasthenia gravis, reversal of NMJ blockade	↑ endogenous ACh; ↑ strength
Physostigmine, echothiophate	Glaucoma	↑ endogenous ACh

(handwritten: PBC – Penn Boys Club)

Antimuscarinic drugs

Organ System	Drugs	Application
CNS	Benztropine	Parkinson's disease
	Scopolamine	Motion sickness
Eye	Atropine, homatropine, tropicamide	Produce mydriasis and cycloplegia
GU	Oxybutynin	Transient cystitis, post-op bladder spasms

HIGH-YIELD FACTS

Pharmacology

Pharmacology

HIGH-YIELD FACTS

Autonomic second messengers

Receptor	Major functions
α_1	↑ Ca^{2+}, causes contraction, secretion
α_2	↓ transmitter release, causes contraction
β_1	↑ heart rate, ↑ contractability; ↑ renin release
β_2	Relaxes smooth muscle; ↑ glycogenolysis; ↑ heart rate, ↑ contractility
β_3	↑ lipolysis
D_1	Relaxes renal vascular smooth muscle

Receptor (M_1, M_3, α_1) $\xrightarrow{G_q}$ Phospholipase C $\longrightarrow$ Lipids ↓ PIP_2 $\rightarrow$ IP_3 $\rightarrow$ ↑ Ca, $\rightarrow$ DAG $\rightarrow$ Protein kinase

Receptor (β, D_1) $\xrightarrow{G_s}$ Adenylylcyclase $\longrightarrow$ ATP ↓ cAMP $\rightarrow$ Channels, Enzymes

Receptor (α_2, M_2) $\xrightarrow{G_i}$ Adenylylcyclase $\longrightarrow$ ↓ cAMP

Sympathomimetics

Drug	Mechanism/Selectivity	Applications
Catecholamines:		
Epinephrine	Direct general agonist $(\alpha_1, \alpha_2, \beta_1, \beta_2)$	Anaphylaxis, glaucoma, asthma, to cause vasoconstriction
Norepinephrine	$\alpha_1, \alpha_2, \beta_1$	To cause vasoconstriction in hypotension
Isoproterenol	$\beta_1 = \beta_2$	Asthma, AV block (rare)
Dopamine	$D_1 = D_2 > \beta > \alpha$	Shock, heart failure
Dobutamine	$\beta_1 > \beta_2$	Shock, heart failure
Other:		
Amphetamine	Indirect general agonist, releases stored catecholamines	Narcolepsy, obesity, attention deficit disorder
Ephedrine	Indirect general agonist, releases stored catecholamines	Nasal congestion, urinary incontinence, to cause vasoconstriction in hypotension
Phenylephrine	$\alpha_1 > \alpha_2$	To cause mydriasis, vasoconstriction, nasal decongestion
Albuterol, terbutaline	$\beta_2 > \beta_1$	Asthma
Cocaine	Indirect general agonist, uptake inhibitor	To cause vasoconstriction and local anesthesia

α Blockers	Application	Toxicity
Nonselective		
Phenoxybenzamine (irreversible)	Pheochromocytoma	Orthostatic hypotension, reflex tachycardia
Phentolamine (reversible)	Pheochromocytoma, impotence	Orthostatic hypotension, reflex tachycardia
α_1-selective		
Prazosin, terazosin	Hypertension, urinary retention in BPH	First-dose orthostatic hypotension (prazosin), dizziness, headache
α_2-selective		
Yohimbine	Impotence	

β Blockers

Propranolol, metoprolol, atenolol, nadolol, timolol, pindolol, esmolol

Application	Effect
Hypertension	↓ cardiac output, ↓ renin secretion
Angina pectoris	↓ heart rate and contractility, resulting in decreased oxygen consumption
SVT (propranolol, esmolol)	↓ AV conduction velocity
Glaucoma (timolol)	↓ secretion of aqueous humor
Toxicity	Impotence, exacerbation of asthma, cardiovascular adverse effects (bradycardia, AV block, CHF), CNS adverse effects (sedation, sleep alterations)

Barbiturates

	Phenobarbital, pentobarbital, thiopental, secobarbital
Mechanism	Facilitate GABA action by ↑ **duration** of Cl⁻ channel opening.
Clinical use	Anxiety, seizures, insomnia, induction of anesthesia (thiopental).
Toxicity	Dependence, additive CNS depression effects with alcohol, respiratory or cardiovascular depression, drug interactions owing to induction of liver microsomal enzymes (cyt. P450).

Benzodiazepines

	Diazepam, lorazepam, triazolam, temazepam, chlordiazepoxide
Mechanism	Facilitates GABA action by ↑ **frequency** of Cl⁻ channel opening. Most have long half-lives and active metabolites.
Clinical use	Anxiety, spasticity, status epilepticus (diazepam), detoxification (especially alcohol).
Toxicity	Dependence, additive CNS depression effects with alcohol. Treat overdose with flumazenil.

Antipsychotics

	Thioridazine, haloperidol, chlorpromazine.	Evolution of EPS side effects:
Mechanism	Most antipsychotics block dopamine D_2 receptors (excess dopamine effects connected with schizophrenia).	4 h acute dystonia
Clinical use	Schizophrenia, psychosis.	4 d akinesia
Toxicity	Extrapyramidal system side effects, sedation, endocrine side effects, and side effects arising from blocking muscarinic, α, and histamine receptors. Retinal deposits from thioridazine. Neuroleptic malignant syndrome: rigidity, autonomic instability, hyperpyrexia.	4 wk akathisia; 4 mo tardive dyskinesia (irreversible).

Pharmacology

HIGH-YIELD FACTS

Clozapine

Mechanism	Atypical—blocks dopamine D_4 receptors.
Clinical use	2nd line drug for treatment of schizophrenia, psychosis.
Toxicity	Less sedation, anticholinergic, and extrapyramidal symptoms than typical antipsychotics. Causes agranulocytosis requiring WBC monitoring.

Lithium

Mechanism	Not established; possibly related to inhibition of phosphoinositol cascade.
Clinical use	Mood stabilizer for bipolar affective disorder, blocks relapse and acute manic events.
Toxicity	Tremor, hypothyroidism, polyuria (ADH antagonist), teratogenesis. Narrow therapeutic window requiring close monitoring of serum levels.

Tricyclic antidepressants

Imipramine, amitriptyline, desipramine, nortriptyline, clomipramine, doxepin

Mechanism	Block reuptake of norepinephrine and serotonin.
Clinical use	Endogenous depression, bedwetting (imipramine), obsessive-compulsive disorder (clomipramine).
Side effects	Sedation, α-blocking effects, atropine-like side effects (tachycardia, urinary retention).
Toxicity	Convulsions, coma, respiratory depression, hyperpyrexia, arrhythmias. Confusion and hallucinations in elderly.

SSRIs

Fluoxetine, sertraline, paroxetine

Mechanism	Serotonin-specific reuptake inhibitors.
Clinical use	Endogenous depression.
Toxicity	Anxiety, insomnia, tremor, anorexia, nausea, and vomiting.

Monoamine oxidase (MAO) inhibitors

Phenelzine, isocarboxazid, tranylcypromine

Mechanism	Nonselective MAO inhibition.
Clinical use	Atypical depressions (i.e., with psychotic or phobic features), anxiety, hypochondriasis.
Toxicity	Hypertensive reactions with tyramine and meperidine; CNS stimulation.

Selegiline

Mechanism	Selectively inhibits MAO-B, thereby increasing the availability of dopamine.
Clinical use	Adjunctive agent to L-dopa in treatment of Parkinson's disease.
Toxicity	May enhance adverse effects of L-dopa.

L-dopa

Mechanism	Increases level of dopamine in brain. Parkinsonism thought to be due to loss of dopaminergic neurons and excess cholinergic function. Unlike dopamine, L-dopa can cross blood-brain barrier and is converted by dopa decarboxylase in the CNS to dopamine.
Clinical use	Parkinsonism.
Toxicity	Dyskinesias, arrhythmias from peripheral conversion to dopamine (carbidopa given with L-dopa inhibits peripheral decarboxylase).

Opioid analgesics

Morphine, codeine, heroin, methadone, meperidine, dextromethorphan

Mechanism	Act as agonists at opioid receptors to modulate synaptic transmission.
Clinical use	Pain, cough suppression, diarrhea, acute pulmonary edema, maintenance programs for addicts (methadone).
Toxicity	Addiction, respiratory depression, constipation, miosis, additive CNS depression with other drugs. Toxicity treated with naloxone (opioid receptor antagonist).

Sumatriptan

Mechanism	5-HT$_{1d}$ agonist. Half-life < 2 hours. Very expensive.
Clinical use	Acute migraine, cluster headache attacks.
Toxicity	Chest discomfort, mild tingling (contraindicated in patients with CAD or Prinzmetal's angina).

Ondansetron

Mechanism	5-HT$_3$ antagonist. Powerful central-acting antiemetic.
Clinical use	Control vomiting postoperatively and in patients undergoing cancer chemotherapy.
Toxicity	Headache, diarrhea.

Epilepsy drugs

Indications	Drugs of choice
Grand mal seizure	Phenytoin, phenobarbital, carbamazepine
Status epilepticus	Diazepam, lorazepam, phenytoin
Complex partial (temporal lobe)	Primidone, carbamazepine
Petit mal (absence)	Ethosuximide, valproic acid, clonazepam
Trigeminal neuralgia	Carbamazepine

Epilepsy drug toxicities

Benzodiazepines	Sedation, tolerance, dependence.
Carbamazepine	Diplopia, ataxia, induction of cyt. P450, blood dyscrasias.
Ethosuximide	Gastrointestinal distress, lethargy, headache.
Phenobarbital	Sedation, induction of cyt. P450, tolerance, dependence.
Phenytoin	Nystagmus, diplopia, ataxia, sedation, gingival hyperplasia, hirsutism, anemias, birth defects (teratogenic).
Valproic acid	Gastrointestinal distress, rare but fatal hepatotoxicity, neural tube defects in fetus.

Phenytoin

Mechanism	Use-dependent blockade of Na$^+$ channels.
Clinical use	Grand mal seizures.
Toxicity	Nystagmus, ataxia, diplopia, lethargy. Chronic use produces gingival hyperplasia in children, peripheral neuropathy, hirsutism, megaloblastic anemia, teratogenic.

Inhaled anesthetics

Halothane, enflurane, isoflurane, seroflurane, methoxyflurane, nitrous oxide

Principle	The lower the solubility, the quicker the anesthetic induction and the quicker the recovery.
Effects	Myocardial depression, respiratory depression, nausea/emesis, ↑ cerebral blood flow.
Toxicity	Hepatotoxicity (halothane), nephrotoxicity (methoxyflurane), proconvulsant (enflurane).

Intravenous anesthetics

Barbiturates	Thiopental: high lipid solubility, rapid entry into brain. Used for induction of anesthesia and short surgical procedures. Effect terminated by redistribution from brain. ↓ cerebral blood flow.
Benzodiazepines	Midazolam: used adjunctively with gaseous anesthetics and narcotics. May cause severe postoperative respiratory depression and amnesia.
Arylcyclohexylamines	Ketamine: dissociative anesthetic. Cardiovascular stimulant. Causes disorientation, hallucination, and bad dreams. Increases cerebral blood flow.
Narcotic analgesics	Morphine, fentanyl: used with other CNS depressants during general anesthesia.
Other	Propofol: used for rapid anesthesia induction and short procedures. Less postop nausea than thiopental.

Local anesthetics

	Procaine, lidocaine, bupivacaine, cocaine
Mechanism	Block Na⁺ channels by binding to specific receptors on inner portion of channel. Tertiary amine local anesthetics penetrate membrane in uncharged form, then bind in charged form.
Principle	1. In infected (acidic) tissue, anesthetics are charged and cannot penetrate membrane effectively. Therefore more anesthetic is needed in these cases.
	2. Small-diameter, myelinated fibers are blocked more easily than large-diameter, unmyelinated ones (sympathetic fibers are blocked 2 levels higher than pain fibers).
	3. Given with vasoconstrictors (usually epinephrine) to enhance local action.
Clinical use	Minor surgical procedures.
Toxicity	CNS excitation, severe cardiovascular toxicity (bupivacaine), hypertension and arrhythmias (cocaine).

Pharmacology

HIGH-YIELD FACTS

Antihypertensive drugs

Drug	Adverse effects
Diuretics	
Hydrochlorothiazide	Hypokalemia, slight hyperlipidemia, hyperuricemia, depression
Sympathoplegics	
Clonidine	Dry mouth, sedation, severe rebound hypertension
Methyldopa	Sedation, positive Coombs' test
Ganglionic blockers	Severe orthostatic hypotension, blurred vision, constipation, sexual dysfunction
Reserpine	Sedation, depression, nasal stuffiness, diarrhea
Guanethidine	Orthostatic and exercise hypotension, sexual dysfunction, diarrhea
Prazosin	First-dose orthostatic hypotension, dizziness, headache
β blockers	Impotence, asthma, CV effects (bradycardia, CHF, AV block), CNS effects (sedation, sleep alterations)
Vasodilators	
Hydralazine	Nausea, headache, lupus-like syndrome, tachycardia, angina, salt retention
Minoxidil	Hirsutism, pericardial effusion, tachycardia, angina, salt retention
Nifedipine	Constipation, nausea, dizziness, flushing
Nitroprusside	Cyanide toxicity (releases CN)
ACE inhibitors	
Captopril	Cough, taste changes, rash, proteinuria, renal damage in fetus

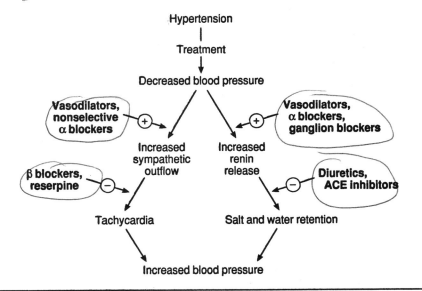

Calcium channel blockers

Nifedipine, verapamil, diltiazem

Mechanism
Block voltage-dependent calcium channels of cardiac and smooth muscle and thereby reduce muscle contractility.
Vascular smooth muscle: nifedipine > diltiazem > verapamil
Heart: verapamil > diltiazem > nifedipine

Clinical use
Hypertension, angina, arrhythmias.

Toxicity
Cardiac depression, peripheral edema, flushing, dizziness, and constipation.

ACE inhibitors

Captopril, enalapril, lisinopril

Mechanism
Inhibit angiotensin-converting enzyme, reducing levels of angiotensin II and preventing inactivation of bradykinin, a potent vasodilator.

Clinical use
Hypertension, congestive heart failure, diabetic renal vascular disease.

Toxicity
Cough, proteinuria, rash, taste changes.

Furosemide

Mechanism
Sulfonamide loop diuretic. Inhibits cotransport system (Na^+, K^+, $2 Cl^-$) of thick ascending limb of loop of Henle. Abolishes hypertonicity of medulla, preventing concentration of urine.

Clinical use
Edematous states (CHF, cirrhosis, nephrotic syndrome, pulmonary edema), HTN, hypercalcemia.

Toxicity
Ototoxicity, **H**ypokalemia, **S**evere dehydration, **H**ypersensitivity (sulfa), **I**nterstitial nephritis, gou**T**.   Toxicity: OH *?@!

Ethacrynic acid

Mechanism
Phenoxyacetic acid derivative (NOT a sulfonamide). Essentially same action as furosemide.

Clinical use
Diuresis in patients allergic to sulfa drugs.

Toxicity
Similar to furosemide except no hyperuricemia, no sulfa allergies.

Hydrochlorothiazide

Mechanism
Thiazide diuretic. Inhibits NaCl reabsorption in early distal tubule, reducing diluting capacity of the nephron.

Clinical use
Hypertension, congestive heart failure, calcium stone formation, nephrogenic diabetes insipidus.

Toxicity
Hypokalemic metabolic alkalosis, hyponatremia, hyperglycemia, hyperlipidemia, and hyperuricemia.

Acetazolamide

Mechanism
Carbonic anhydrase inhibitor. Causes self-limited $NaHCO_3$ diuresis and reduction in total-body HCO_3^- stores. Acts at the proximal convoluted tubule.

Clinical use
Glaucoma, urinary alkalinization, metabolic alkalosis.

Toxicity
Hyperchloremic metabolic acidosis, neuropathy, NH_3 toxicity.

Spironolactone

Mechanism	Competitive antagonist to aldosterone, K^+-sparing diuretic.
Clinical use	Hyperaldosteronism, K^+ depletion.
Toxicity	Hyperkalemia, endocrine effects (gynecomastia, antiandrogen effects).

Diuretics: electrolyte changes

Urine NaCl	↑ (All diuretics: Carbonic anhydrase inhibitors, loop diuretics, thiazides, K^+-sparing diuretics)
Urine K^+	↑ (All except K^+-sparing diuretics)
Blood pH	↓ (acidosis): CA inhibitors, K^+-sparing diuretics
	↑ (alkalosis): Loop diuretics, thiazides

Diuretics: site of action

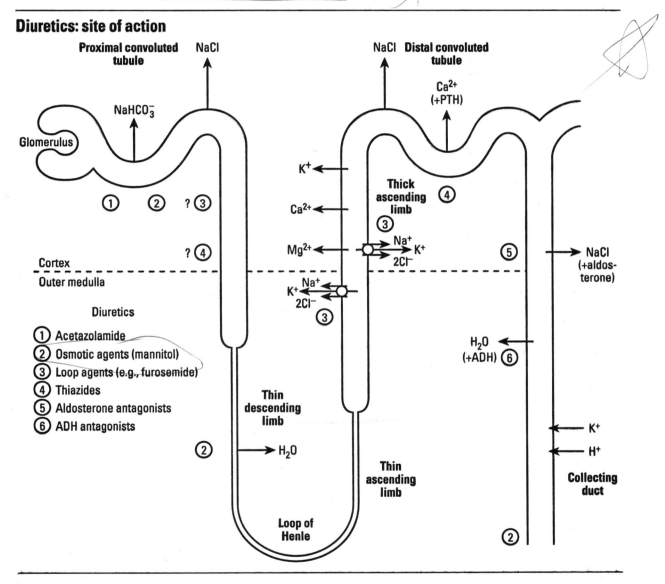

Diuretics
1. Acetazolamide
2. Osmotic agents (mannitol)
3. Loop agents (e.g., furosemide)
4. Thiazides
5. Aldosterone antagonists
6. ADH antagonists

Nitroglycerin, isosorbide dinitrate

Mechanism	Vasodilate by releasing nitric oxide in smooth muscle, causing increase in cGMP and smooth muscle relaxation.
Clinical use	Angina, pulmonary edema. Also used as an aphrodisiac and erection-enhancer.
Toxicity	Tachycardia, hypotension, headache, "Monday disease" in industrial exposure (alternating development of tolerance during the work week and loss of tolerance over the weekend for the vasodilating action, resulting in tachycardia, dizziness, and headache every Monday).

Cardiac glycosides

Digoxin: 75% bioavailability, 20–40% protein bound, $T_{1/2} = 40$ hr, urinary excretion

Digitoxin: > 95% bioavailability, 70% protein bound, $T_{1/2} = 168$ hrs, biliary excretion (enterohepatic recycling)

Mechanism	Inhibits the Na^+-K^+-ATPase of cell membrane, causing ↑ intracellular Na^+. Na^+-Ca^{2+} antiport does not function as efficiently, causing ↑ intracellular Ca^{2+}; leads to positive inotropy.
Clinical use	CHF, atrial fibrillation.
Toxicity	Nausea, vomiting, diarrhea. Yellowing of vision. Gynecomastia. Arrhythmia: Early ECG changes—↑ PR interval, bradycardia, flattened T wave. Later ECG changes—inverted T wave, ST depression, decreased QT. Late ECG changes—↑ automaticity, delayed afterdepolarizations, bigeminy, PVCs, fibrillation.
Antidote	Slowly normalize K^+, lidocaine, cardiac pacer, anti-dig Fab fragments.

Antiarrhythmics—Na⁺ channel blockers

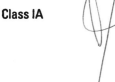

Local anesthetics. Slow or block (↓) conduction (especially in depolarized cells) and ↓ abnormal pacemakers that are Na⁺ channel dependent. Are state dependent (i.e., selectively depress tissue that is frequently depolarized, e.g., fast tachycardia).

Class IA
Quinidine, amiodarone, procainamide, disopyramide.

↑ AP duration, ↑ effective refractory period (ERP), ↑ QT interval. Affect both atrial and ventricular arrhythmias.

Toxicity: Quinidine (cinchonism: headache, tinnitus; thrombocytopenia, torsade de pointes); procainamide (reversible SLE-like syndrome).

Class IB
Lidocaine, mexiletine, tocainide.

↓ AP duration. Affect ischemic or depolarized Purkinje and ventricular tissue. Useful in acute ventricular arrhythmias (especially post-MI), and in digitalis-induced arrhythmias.

Toxicity: Local anesthetic toxicity (CNS stimulation/depression, cardiovascular depression).

Class IC
Flecainide, encainide, propafenone.

No effect on AP duration. Useful in V-tachs that progress to VF, and in intractable SVT. Are usually used only as last resort in refractory tachyarrhythmias because of toxicities.

Toxicity: Proarrhythmic, CNS stimulation.

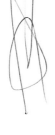

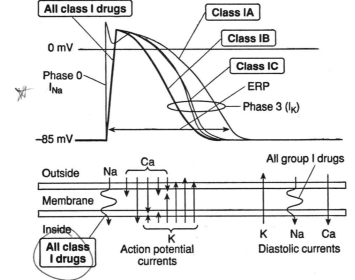

Antiarrhythmics—β blockers

Propranolol, esmolol, metoprolol, timolol.
↓ cAMP, ↓Ca²⁺ currents. Suppress abnormal
pacemakers. AV node particularly sensitive: ↑ PR
interval. Esmolol very short-acting.
Toxicity: Impotence, exacerbation of asthma, CV effects
(bradycardia, AV block, CHF), CNS effects (sedation,
sleep alterations).

Antiarrhythmics—K⁺ channel blockers

Sotalol, bretylium, amiodarone.
↑ AP duration, ↑ ERP. Bretylium is rarely used, and only in post-MI arrhythmias
(e.g., recurrent VF).
Toxicity: Sotalol (torsade de pointes, excessive β block).
Bretylium (new arrhythmias, hypotension).
Amiodarone (pulmonary fibrosis, corneal deposits, skin deposits resulting in
photodermatitis, neurologic effects, constipation, CV effects (bradycardia, heart block,
CHF), hypo/hyperthyroidism.

Amy:
Lungs, Eyes,
Skin, Nerve

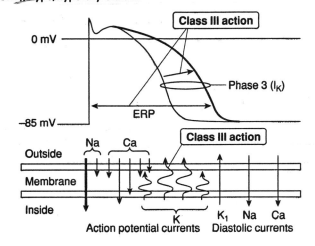

Antiarrhythmics—Ca²⁺ channel blockers

Verapamil, diltiazem, bepridil.

↓ conduction velocity, ↑ ERP, ↑ PR interval. Used in prevention of nodal arrhythmias (e.g., SVT).

Toxicity: Constipation, flushing, edema, nausea, CV effects (CHF, AV block, sinus node depression).

Bepridil (torsade de pointes).

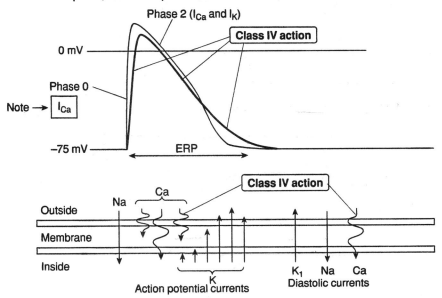

Antiarrhythmics—Miscellaneous

Adenosine	Drug of choice in abolishing AV nodal arrhythmias.
K⁺	Depresses ectopic pacemakers, especially in digoxin toxicity.
Mg⁺	Effective in torsade de pointes and digoxin toxicity.

PHARMACOLOGY—CANCER DRUGS

Cyclophosphamide

Mechanism	Alkylating agent; covalently x-links (interstrand) DNA at guanine N-7. Requires bioactivation by liver.
Clinical use	Non-Hodgkin's lymphoma, breast and ovarian carcinomas.
Toxicity	Myelosuppression, hemorrhagic cystitis. → MESNA

Cisplatin

Mechanism	Acts like an alkylating agent. X-links via hydrolysis of Cl⁻ groups and reaction with platinum.
Clinical use	Testicular and lung carcinomas.
Toxicity	Nephrotoxicity and acoustic nerve damage.

Doxorubicin (adriamycin)

Mechanism	Anthracycline antibiotic; noncovalently intercalates in DNA to decrease replication and transcription and generate free radicals.
Clinical use	Part of the ABVD combo regimen for myelomas, sarcomas, and lymphomas.
Toxicity	Cardiotoxicity; also myelosuppression and marked alopecia.

Methotrexate

Mechanism	S-phase specific antimetabolite. Folic acid analog that inhibits dihydrofolate reductase, resulting in decreased dTMP and therefore decreased DNA and protein synthesis.
Clinical use	Leukemias, sarcomas, abortion, ectopic pregnancy, rheumatoid arthritis.
Toxicity	Myelosuppression, which is reversible with leukovorin "rescue."

5-fluorouracil (5-FU)

Mechanism	S-phase-specific antimetabolite. Pyrimidine analog bioactivated to 5FdUMP, which covalently complexes folic acid. This complex inhibits thymidylate synthase, resulting in decreased dTMP and same effects as methotrexate.
Clinical use	Colon cancer, basal cell carcinoma (topical).
Toxicity	Myelosuppression, which is NOT reversible with leukovorin; photosensitivity.

Vincristine and vinblastine

Mechanism	M-phase-specific alkaloid from the periwinkle plant (*Vinca rosea*) that binds to tubulin and blocks polymerization of microtubules so that mitotic spindle can't form.
Clinical use	Part of MOPP (Oncovin) combo regimen for lymphoma, Wilms' tumor, choriocarcinoma.
Toxicity	Vincristine—Neurotoxicity (areflexia, peripheral neuritis), paralytic ileus. Vinblastine causes bone marrow suppression.

Taxol

Mechanism	M-phase-specific agent obtained from yew tree that binds to tubulin and hyperstabilizes polymerized microtubules so that mitotic spindle can't break down (anaphase cannot occur).
Clinical use	Ovarian and breast carcinomas.
Toxicity	Myelosuppression and cardiotoxicity.

Etoposide

Mechanism	G_2-phase-specific podophyllotoxin that inhibits topoisomerase II so that double-strand breaks remain in DNA following replication, with subsequent DNA degradation.
Clinical use	Oat cell carcinoma of the lung and prostate, testicular carcinoma.
Toxicity	Myelosuppression, GI irritation, alopecia.

Prednisone

Mechanism	May trigger apoptosis. May even work on non-growth fraction cells.
Clinical use	Most commonly used glucocorticoid in cancer chemotherapy. Used in CLL, Hodgkin's lymphomas, rheumatoid arthritis, asthma.
Toxicity	Cushing-like symptoms; immunosuppression.

Tamoxifen

Mechanism	Estrogen receptor mixed agonist/antagonist that blocks the binding of estrogen to ER+ cells.
Clinical use	Breast cancer.
Toxicity	May increase the risk of endometrial carcinoma via partial agonist effects; "hot flashes."

PHARMACOLOGY—TOXICOLOGY

Specific antidotes

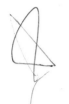

Toxin	Antidote/treatment
1. Acetaminophen	1. N-acetylcysteine - Mucomyst
2. Anticholinesterases, organophosphates	2. Atropine, pralidoxime
3. Iron salts	3. Deferoxamine
4. Methanol, ethylene glycol (antifreeze)	4. Ethanol, dialysis
5. Lead	5. CaEDTA, dimercaprol
6. Arsenic, mercury, gold	6. Dimercaprol (BAL)
7. Copper, arsenic, lead, gold	7. Penicillamine
8. Antimuscarinic, anticholinergic agents	8. Physostigmine salicylate
9. Cyanide	9. Nitrite
10. Salicylates	10. Alkalinize urine, dialysis
11. Heparin	11. Protamine
12. Methemoglobinemia	12. Methylene blue
13. Opioids	13. Naloxone
14. Benzodiazepines	14. Flumazenil
15. Tricyclic antidepressant arrhythmias	15. NaHCO$_3$
16. Warfarin	16. Vitamin K$^+$, FFP
17. Carbon monoxide	17. 100% O$_2$, hyperbaric O$_2$
18. Digitalis	18. Stop dig, normalize K$^+$, lidocaine, anti-dig Fab fragments
19. β blockers	19. Glucagon
20. t-PA, streptokinase	20. Aminocaproic acid
21. PCP	21. Nasogastric suction

Lead poisoning

Lead Lines on gingivae, and on epiphysis of long bones on x-ray. **LEAD**

Encephalopathy and Erythrocyte basophilic stippling.

Abdominal colic and sideroblastic Anemia.

Drops: wrist and foot drop. Dimercaprol and EDTA as first line of treatment.

Urine pH and drug elimination

Weak acids (phenobarbital, methotrexate, aspirin) ⇒ alkalinize urine

Weak bases (amphetamines) ⇒ acidify urine.

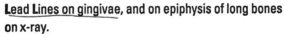

Drug reactions

Drug reaction	Causal agent
1. Pulmonary fibrosis	1. Bleomycin, amiodarone
2. Hepatitis	2. Isoniazid (INH)
3. Focal to massive hepatic necrosis	3. Halothane
4. Anaphylaxis	4. Penicillin
5. SLE-like syndrome	5. Hydralazine, procainamide
6. Blood dyscrasias	6. Ibuprofen, quinidine, methyldopa, chemotherapy
7. Hemolysis in G6PD-deficient patients	7. Sulfonamides, INH, aspirin, ibuprofen, primaquine
8. Benign and malignant proliferations	8. Estrogens
9. Thrombotic complications	9. Oral contraceptives (e.g., estrogens and progestins)
10. Adrenocortical insufficiency	10. Glucocorticoids
11. Photosensitivity reactions	11. Tetracyclines, amiodarone, sulfonamides
12. Gynecomastia	12. Cimetidine, ketoconazole, spironolactone
13. Induce ($\uparrow$) P450 system	13. Barbiturates, phenytoin, carbamazapine, rifampin
14. Inhibit ($\downarrow$) P450 system	14. Cimetidine, ketoconazole
15. Tubulointerstitial nephritis	15. Sulfonamides
16. Teratogenic effects	16. Ethanol, lithium, warfarin, valproic acid, thalidomide, isotretinoin, androgens
17. Carcinogenic effects	17. Aflatoxin, vinyl chloride, coal tar, polycyclic aromatic hydrocarbons (in tobacco smoke)
18. Mutagenic effects	18. Aflatoxin, cancer chemotherapeutic drugs
19. Hot flashes	19. Tamoxifen
20. Cutaneous flushing	20. Niacin, Ca^{2+} channel blockers

Pharmacology

HIGH-YIELD FACTS

Alcohol toxicity

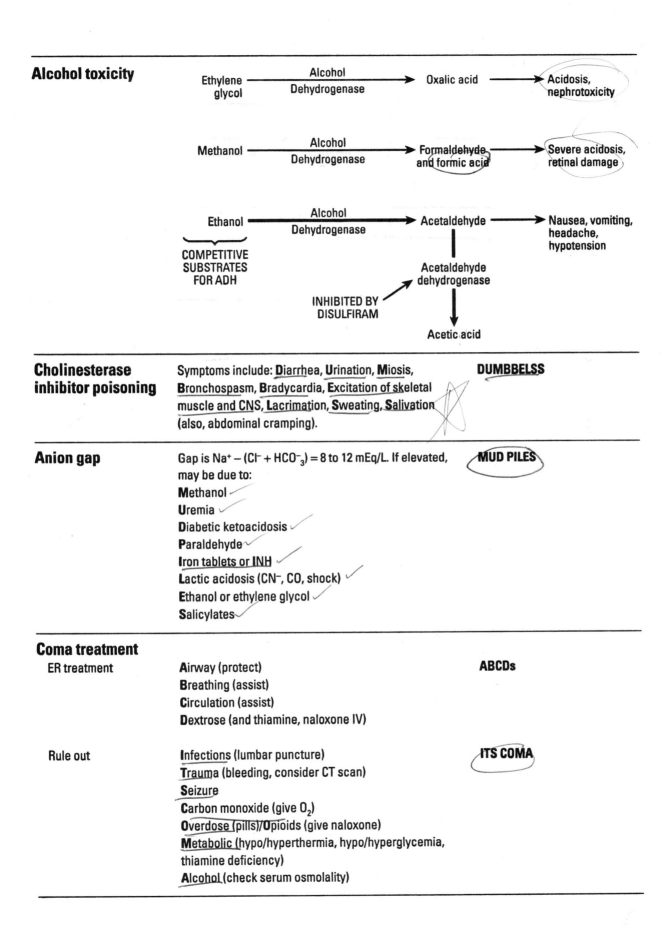

Ethylene glycol → (Alcohol Dehydrogenase) → Oxalic acid → Acidosis, nephrotoxicity

Methanol → (Alcohol Dehydrogenase) → Formaldehyde and formic acid → Severe acidosis, retinal damage

Ethanol → (Alcohol Dehydrogenase) → Acetaldehyde → Nausea, vomiting, headache, hypotension

COMPETITIVE SUBSTRATES FOR ADH

Acetaldehyde → (Acetaldehyde dehydrogenase) → Acetic acid

INHIBITED BY DISULFIRAM

Cholinesterase inhibitor poisoning

Symptoms include: **D**iarrhea, **U**rination, **M**iosis, **B**ronchospasm, **B**radycardia, **E**xcitation of skeletal muscle and CNS, **L**acrimation, **S**weating, **S**alivation (also, abdominal cramping).

DUMBBELSS

Anion gap

Gap is $Na^+ - (Cl^- + HCO_3^-) = 8$ to 12 mEq/L. If elevated, may be due to:

Methanol
Uremia
Diabetic ketoacidosis
Paraldehyde
Iron tablets or INH
Lactic acidosis (CN^-, CO, shock)
Ethanol or ethylene glycol
Salicylates

MUD PILES

Coma treatment

ER treatment

Airway (protect)
Breathing (assist)
Circulation (assist)
Dextrose (and thiamine, naloxone IV)

ABCDs

Rule out

Infections (lumbar puncture)
Trauma (bleeding, consider CT scan)
Seizure
Carbon monoxide (give O_2)
Overdose (pills)/**O**pioids (give naloxone)
Metabolic (hypo/hyperthermia, hypo/hyperglycemia, thiamine deficiency)
Alcohol (check serum osmolality)

ITS COMA

H$_2$ blockers

Cimetidine, ranitidine, famotidine

Mechanism	Reversible block of histamine H$_2$ receptors.
Clinical use	Peptic ulcer, gastritis, esophageal reflux, Zollinger-Ellison syndrome.
Toxicity	Cimetidine is a potent inhibitor of hepatic drug-metabolizing enzymes, it also has an antiandrogen effect. Other H$_2$ blockers are relatively free of these effects.

Omeprazole

Mechanism	Irreversibly inhibits H$^+$/K$^+$ ATPase in stomach cells.
Clinical use	Peptic ulcer, gastritis, esophageal reflux, Zollinger-Ellison syndrome.

Sucralfate

Mechanism	Aluminum sucrose sulfate polymerizes in the acid environment of the stomach and selectively binds necrotic peptic ulcer tissue. Acts as a barrier to acid, pepsin, and bile. Sucralfate cannot work in the presence of antacids or H$_2$ blockers (requires acidic environment to polymerize).
Clinical use	Peptic ulcer disease.
Toxicity	GI upset (minor and rare).

Misoprostol

Mechanism	A PGE$_1$ analog. Increases production and secretion of gastric mucous barrier.
Clinical use	Prevention of NSAID-induced peptic ulcers.
Toxicity	Diarrhea. Contraindicated in women of childbearing potential (abortifacient).

Heparin

Mechanism	Catalyzes the activation of antithrombin III. Short half-life.
Clinical use	Immediate anticoagulation, used in pregnancy (doesn't cross placenta).
Toxicity	Bleeding, thrombocytopenia, drug-drug interactions. Use protamine sulfate for rapid reversal of heparinization.

Warfarin (Coumadin)

Mechanism	Interferes with normal synthesis of vit. K-dependent clotting factors II, VII, IX, and X via vitamin K antagonism. Long half-life.
Clinical use	Chronic anticoagulation except in pregnant women (since warfarin, unlike heparin, can cross the placenta).
Toxicity	Bleeding, teratogen, drug-drug interactions.

Named after the **W**isconsin **A**lumni **R**esearch **F**oundation (useless but true).

Heparin vs. warfarin

	Heparin	Warfarin
Structure	Large anionic polymer, acidic	Small lipid-soluble molecule
Route of administration	Parenteral (IV, SC)	Oral
Site of action	Blood	Liver
Onset of action	Rapid (seconds)	Slow, limited by half-lives of normal clotting factors
Mechanism of action	Activates antithrombin III	Impairs the synthesis of vit. K-dependent clotting factors II, VII, IX, and X (vit. K antagonist)
Duration of action	Acute (days)	Chronic (weeks or months)
Inhibits coagulation *in vitro*	Yes	No
Treatment of acute overdose	Protamine sulfate	IV vit. K and fresh frozen plasma

Thrombolytics

	Streptokinase, urokinase, tPA (alteplase), APSAC (anistreplase)	tPA: human protein produced in bacteria.
Mechanism	Directly or indirectly aid conversion of plasminogen to plasmin.	Urokinase: from cultured human kidney cells.
Clinical use	Early myocardial infarction.	Streptokinase: from bacteria.
Toxicity	Bleeding.	APSAC: prodrug made of streptokinase plus recombinant human plasminogen.

Cholinoreceptor blockers

Muscarinic antagonists	Atropine: used to dilate pupil, reduce acid secretion in acid-peptic disease, reduce urgency in mild cystitis, reduce airway secretions. Causes increased body temperature, rapid pulse, dry mouth, flushed skin, disorientation, mydriasis with cycloplegia.	Atropine parasympathetic block effects:
Nicotinic antagonists	Hexamethonium: ganglionic blocker.	Red as a beet
Cholinesterase regenerator	Pralidoxime: regenerates active cholinesterase, chemical antagonist, used to treat organophosphate exposure.	Mad as a hatter Hot as a hare Dry as a bone Bloated as a bladder

Neuromuscular blocking drugs

Depolarizing

Succinylcholine

Reversal of blockade: Phase I—No antidote. Block potentiated by cholinesterase inhibitors
Phase II—Cholinesterase inhibitors (e.g., neostigmine).

Nondepolarizing

Tubocurarine, atracurium, mivacurium, pancuronium, vecuronium.

Reversal of blockade: Neostigmine, edrophonium, and other cholinesterase inhibitors.

Dantrolene

Used in the treatment of malignant hyperthermia, which is caused by the concomitant use of halothane and succinylcholine.

Mechanism: Prevents the release of Ca^{2+} from the sarcoplasmic reticulum of skeletal muscle.

Ritodrine, terbutaline

β_2 agonists used to delay labor by inhibiting uterine smooth muscle contraction.

Asthma drugs

Nonspecific β agonists   Isoproterenol: relaxes bronchial smooth muscle (β_2). Adverse effect is tachycardia (β_1).

β₂ agonists   Albuterol: relaxes bronchial smooth muscle (β_2). Adverse effects are tremor and arrhythmia.

Methylxanthines   Theophylline: mechanism unclear—may cause bronchodilation by inhibiting phosphodiesterase, enzyme involved in degrading cAMP (controversial).

Muscarinic antagonists   Ipratropium: competitive block of muscarinic receptors preventing bronchoconstriction.

Cromolyn   Prevents release of mediators from mast cells. Effective only for the prophylaxis of asthma. Not effective during an active asthmatic attack.

Corticosteroids   Block synthesis of leukotrienes from arachidonic acid by phospholipase A_2. Are drugs of choice in a patient with status asthmaticus.

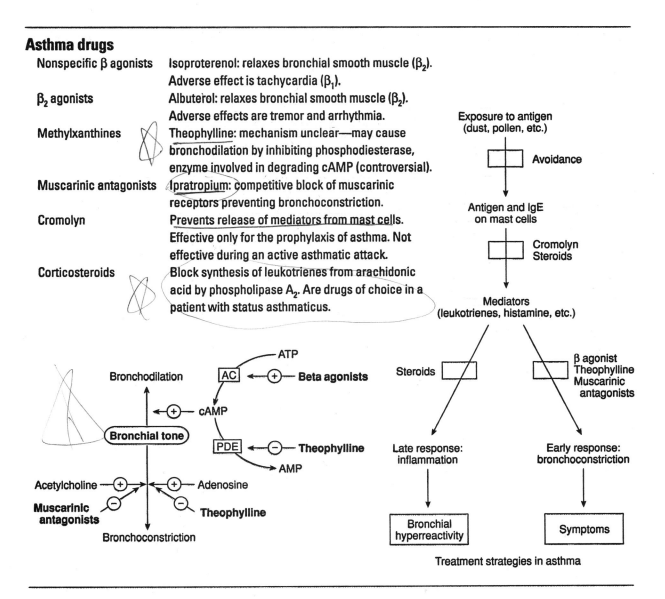

Treatment strategies in asthma

Aspirin

Mechanism	Acetylates and irreversibly inhibits cyclooxygenase to prevent conversion of arachidonic acid to prostaglandins.
Clinical use	Antipyretic, analgesic, anti-inflammatory, antiplatelet drug.
Toxicity	Gastric ulceration, bleeding, hyperventilation, Reye's syndrome, tinnitus, and dizziness (CN VIII).

NSAIDs

Ibuprofen, naproxen, indomethacin

Mechanism	Reversibly inhibit cyclooxygenase.
Clinical use	Antipyretic, analgesic, anti-inflammatory. Indomethacin is used to close a patent ductus arteriosus.
Toxicity	Renal damage, aplastic anemia.

Acetaminophen

Mechanism	Weak prostaglandin inhibitor.
Clinical use	Antipyretic, analgesic, but lacking anti-inflammatory properties.
Toxicity	Overdose produces hepatic necrosis.

Glucocorticoids

Hydrocortisone, prednisone, triamcinolone, dexamethasone

Mechanism	Decrease the production of leukotrienes and prostaglandins from arachidonic acid by inhibiting phospholipase A_2.
Clinical use	Addison's disease, inflammation, and immune suppression.
Toxicity	Iatrogenic Cushing's syndrome: buffalo hump, moon facies, truncal obesity, muscle wasting, thin skin, easy bruisability, osteoporosis, adrenal cortical atrophy, peptic ulcers.

Arachidonic acid products

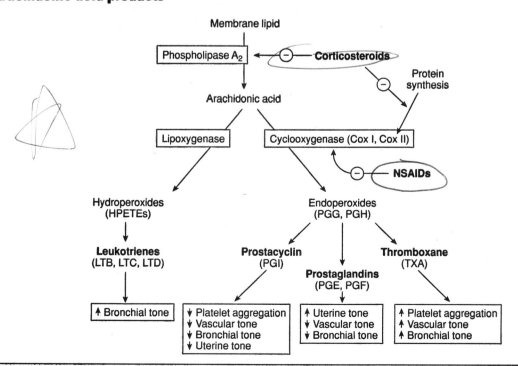

Gout drugs

Colchicine	Acute gout. Depolymerizes microtubules, impairing leukocyte chemotaxis and degranulation. GI side effects, especially if given orally.
Probenecid	Chronic gout. Inhibits reabsorption of uric acid (also inhibits secretion of penicillin).
Allopurinol	Chronic gout. Inhibits xanthine oxidase, decreasing conversion of xanthine to uric acid.

Sulfonylureas

	Tolbutamide, chlorpropamide, glyburide, glipizide.
Mechanism	Oral hypoglycemic agents used to stimulate release of endogenous insulin. Close K⁺ channels in β cell membrane: cell depolarizes, insulin release triggered. Inactive in insulin-dependent diabetics; requires islet cell function.
Clinical use	Non-insulin-dependent (type II) diabetes mellitus.
Toxicity	Hypoglycemia (more common with 2nd generation drugs: glyburide, glipizide). Disulfiram-like effects (not seen with 2nd generation drugs: glyburide, glipizide).

Cholesterol-lowering drugs

Groups	Examples	Toxicities
Bile acid sequestrants	Cholestyramine, colestipol	Bloating, constipation
HMG-CoA reductase inhibitors	Lovastatin, pravastatin	Elevated LFTs, muscle pain
Lipoprotein lipase stimulators	Gemfibrozil, clofibrate	Myalgia, elevated LFTs
VLDL reducers	Niacin	Skin flushing, hyperuricemia
Other	Probucol	Cardiac arrhythmias

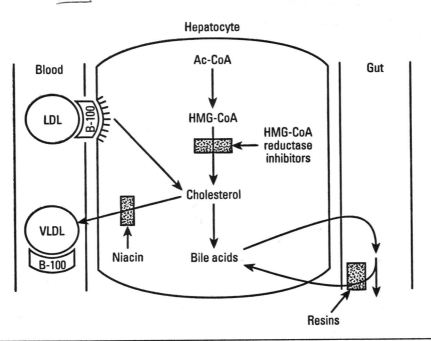

Leuprolide

Mechanism	GnRH analog with agonist properties when used in pulsatile fashion and antagonist properties when used in continuous fashion.
Clinical use	Infertility (pulsatile), prostate cancer (continuous).
Toxicity	Antiandrogen, nausea, vomiting.

Propylthiouracil

Mechanism	Reduces iodination of tyrosine in thyroid (organification).
Clinical use	Hyperthyroidism.
Toxicity	Skin rash, agranulocytosis (rare).

Vasoactive peptides

Angiotensin II (AII)	$\uparrow IP_3$, DAG. Constricts arterioles, $\uparrow$ aldosterone secretion. Also acts at the level of the hypothalamus to increase thirst.
Atrial natriuretic peptide (ANP)	$\uparrow$ cGMP. Dilates vessels, $\downarrow$ aldosterone secretion and effects, $\uparrow$ GFR.

Antiandrogens

Finasteride	A 5α-reductase inhibitor ($\downarrow$ conversion of testosterone to dihydrotestosterone). Useful in BPH.
Flutamide	A nonsteroidal competitive inhibitor of androgens at the testosterone receptor. Used in prostate carcinoma.
Leuprolide	A GnRH analog. Used in prostate cancer, infertility, and uterine fibroids.
Ketoconazole, spironolactone	Inhibit steroid synthesis, used in the treatment of polycystic ovarian syndrome to prevent hirsutism.

Open-angle glaucoma drugs

	Mechanism
Cholinomimetics	Ciliary muscle contraction, opening of trabecular meshwork; $\uparrow$ outflow of aqueous humor
Pilocarpine, carbachol, physostigmine, echothiophate	
α agonists	
Epinephrine	$\uparrow$ outflow of aqueous humor
β blockers	
Timolol, betaxolol, carteolol	$\downarrow$ aqueous humor secretion
Diuretics	
Acetazolamide	$\downarrow$ aqueous humor secretion due to lack of HCO_3^-

Parkinson's disease drugs

Dopamine agonists	L-dopa, bromocriptine (an ergot alkaloid and partial dopamine agonist), amantadine (enhance dopamine release)
MAO inhibitors	Selegiline (selective MAO type B inhibitor)
Antimuscarinics	Benztropine (improve tremor and rigidity but have little effect on bradykinesia)

Nonsurgical antimicrobial prophylaxis

Meningococcal infection	Rifampin (drug of choice), minocycline
Gonorrhea	Ceftriaxone
Syphilis	Benzathine penicillin G
History of recurrent UTI	Trimethoprim-sulfamethoxazole (TMP-SMZ)
PCP	TMP-SMZ (drug of choice), aerosolized pentamidine

Drug development and testing

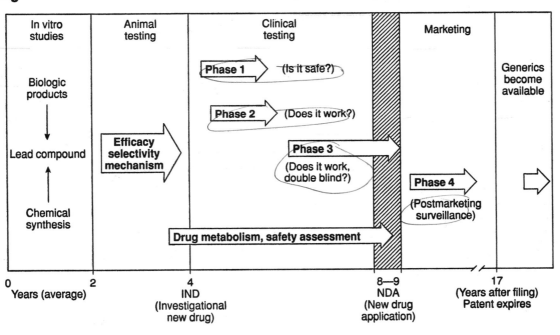

Pharmacokinetics

Volume of distribution (V_d)	Relates the amount of drug in the body to the plasma concentration. V_d of plasma protein-bound drugs can be altered by liver and kidney disease.

$$V_d = \frac{\text{amount of drug in the body}}{\text{plasma drug concentration}}$$

Clearance (CL)	Relates the rate of elimination to the plasma concentration.

$$CL = \frac{\text{rate of elimination of drug}}{\text{plasma drug concentration}}$$

Half-life ($t_{1/2}$)	The time required to change the amount of drug in the body by one-half during elimination (or during a constant infusion). A drug infused at a constant rate reaches 94% of steady state after four $t_{1/2}$.

$$t_{1/2} = \frac{0.7 \times V_d}{CL}$$

Dosage calculations

$$\text{Loading dose} = C_p \times V_d$$
$$\text{Maintenance dose} = C_p \times CL$$
where C_p = target plasma concentration

In patients with impaired renal or hepatic function, the loading dose remains unchanged, while the maintenance dose is decreased

Elimination of drugs

Zero-order elimination	Rate of elimination is constant regardless of C_p. C_p decreases linearly with time. Examples of drugs: ethanol, and phenytoin and aspirin (at high or toxic concentrations).
First-order elimination	Rate of elimination is proportional to the drug concentration. Drug's concentration in plasma (C_p) decreases exponentially with time.

Phase I versus II metabolism

Phase I (reduction, oxidation, hydrolysis) yields slightly polar, water-soluble metabolites (often still active).
Phase II (acetylation, glucuronidation, sulfation) yields very polar inactive metabolites (renally excreted).

Phase I: P450
Phase II: conjugation. Geriatric patients lose phase I first.

Mechanism, clinical use, and toxicity of:

1. Motion sickness drugs (e.g., scopolamine).
2. Antipsychotics, low and high potency.
3. Cholinoceptor-activating drugs (e.g., acetylcholine).
4. Cholinesterase-inhibiting drugs (e.g., neostigmine, edrophonium, physostigmine).
5. Adrenergic drugs (e.g., tyramine).
6. Anti-Parkinsonism drugs (e.g., levodopa, selegiline).
7. Opioid properties (e.g., analgesic, antidiarrheal, antitussive).
8. Immunosuppressive agents (e.g., cyclosporine, azothioprine, corticosteroids).
9. New pharmacologic agents (e.g., sumatriptan, RU486).
10. Myasthenia gravis drugs.

Know about:

1. Complications of empiric antibiotic use (e.g., resistant organisms, fungal infection, pseudomembranous colitis).
2. Secondary effects of common drugs (e.g., heparin: osteoporosis, thiazides: ↑ lipids).
3. Common drugs that enhance/inhibit drug metabolism (e.g., phenobarbital, rifampin, phenytoin, ethanol, cimetidine).
4. Differences between barbiturates and benzodiazepines.
5. Fundamental pharmacokinetics (e.g., half-life, clearance, steady state, volume of distribution).
6. Fundamental pharmacodynamics (e.g., partial agonists, physiologic antagonists, efficacy).
7. Drug efficacy and potency as demonstrated on dose-response curves.
8. Drugs whose metabolism is affected by genetics (e.g., procainamide in slow acetylators).
9. Toxicity and withdrawal symptoms of commonly abused drugs (e.g., heroin, alcohol, cocaine).
10. The physical properties (e.g., MAC, blood:gas partition coefficient) of common anesthetic agents.

HIGH-YIELD FACTS

Pharmacology

Physiology

The portion of the examination dealing with physiology is broad and concept oriented and does not lend itself as well to fact-based review. Diagrams are often the best study aids from which to learn. It may be useful to get help (tutor or group study) if you are weak with basic concepts, as they may be hard to learn from books. Learn to work with basic physiologic relationships in a variety of ways (e.g., Fick equation, clearance equations). You are seldom asked to perform complex calculations. Hormones are the focus of many questions. Learn their sites of production and action as well as their regulatory mechanisms.

A large portion of the physiology tested on the USMLE Step 1 is now clinically relevant and involves understanding of physiologic changes associated with pathologic processes (e.g., changes in pulmonary function testing with chronic obstructive pulmonary disease). Thus, it is worthwhile to review the physiologic changes that are found with common pathologies of the major organ systems (e.g., heart, lungs, kidneys, and gastrointestinal tract).

Cardiovascular
Respiratory
Gastrointestinal
Renal
Endocrine
High-Yield Topics

Myocardial action potential

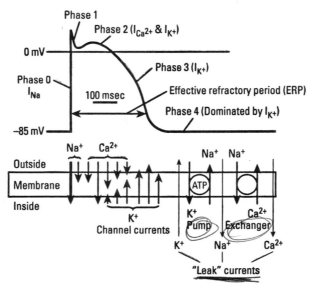

Occurs in atrial and ventricular myocytes and Purkinje fibers.

Phase 0 = Rapid upstroke—voltage-gated Na$^+$ channels open.

Phase 1 = Partial repolarization—inactivation of voltage-gated Na$^+$ channels. Voltage-gated K$^+$ channels begin to open.

Phase 2 = Plateau—Ca^{2+} influx from voltage-gated Ca^{2+} channels balances K$^+$ efflux. Ca^{2+} influx triggers myocyte contraction.

Phase 3 = Rapid repolarization—massive K$^+$ efflux due to opening of voltage-gated slow K$^+$ channels and closure of voltage-gated Ca^{2+} channels.

Phase 4 = Resting potential—high K$^+$ permeability through K1 channels.

Cardiac output

Fick principle:

Cardiac output = (stroke volume) × (heart rate)

$$CO = \frac{\text{Rate of O}_2 \text{ consumption}}{\text{Arterial O}_2 \text{ content} - \text{Venous O}_2 \text{ content}}$$

$$\begin{pmatrix} \text{Mean arterial} \\ \text{pressure} \end{pmatrix} = \begin{pmatrix} \text{cardiac} \\ \text{output} \end{pmatrix} \times \begin{pmatrix} \text{total peripheral} \\ \text{resistance} \end{pmatrix}$$

During exercise, CO increases primarily as a result of increased HR. If HR is too high, the CO drops (e.g., ventricular tachycardia).

Physiology

HIGH-YIELD FACTS

Cardiac output variables

Stroke volume affected by **C**ontractility, **A**fterload, and **P**reload.

Contractility (and SV) increased with:
1. Catecholamines
2. ↑ extracellular calcium
3. ↓ extracellular sodium
4. Digitalis

Contractility (and SV) decreased with:
1. β₁ blockade
2. Heart failure
3. Acidosis
4. Hypoxia/hypercapnea

"SV **CAP**"

Stroke volume increases in anxiety, exercise, and pregnancy.
Pulse pressure is proportional to stroke volume.

A failing heart has decreased stroke volume.
Myocardial O_2 demand is proportional to the heart rate × afterload. Afterload is proportional to the diastolic blood pressure.

Pacemaker action potential

Occurs in the SA and AV nodes. Key differences from the myocardial action potential include:

Phase 0 = slow upstroke—opening of voltage-gated Ca^{2+} channels. These cells lack fast voltage-gated Na^+ channels. Results in a slow conduction velocity that is utilized by the AV node to prolong transmission from the atria to ventricles.

Phase 4 = diastolic depolarization—membrane potential spontaneously depolarizes as K^+ permeability decreases. Rate of diastolic depolarization in the SA node determines heart rate. Acetylcholine decreases and catecholamines increase the slope of this phase, thus decreasing or increasing heart rate, respectively.

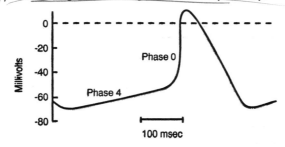

Preload and afterload

Preload = ventricular EDV.
Afterload = peripheral resistance.
Venous dilators (e.g., nitroglycerin) decrease preload.
Vasodilators (e.g., hydralazine) decrease afterload.
↑ SV when ↑ preload or ↓ afterload.

Preload increases with exercise (slightly), extra blood (overtransfusion), and excitement (sympathetics).
Preload pumps up the heart.

Starling curve

Energy of contraction is proportional to initial length of cardiac muscle fiber (preload).

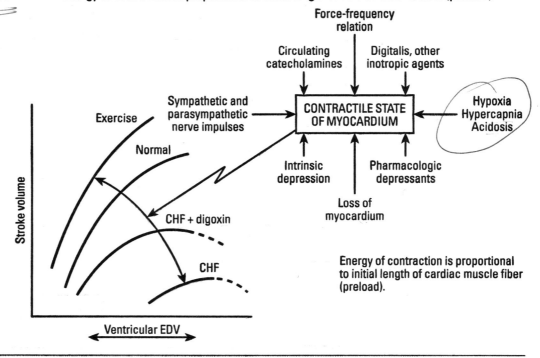

Energy of contraction is proportional to initial length of cardiac muscle fiber (preload).

Ejection fraction

$$\text{Ejection fraction} = \frac{\text{end-diastolic volume} - \text{end-systolic volume}}{\text{end-diastolic volume}}$$

Ejection fraction is an index of ventricular function.

Ejection fraction is normally 60–80%.

Resistance, pressure, flow

$$\text{Resistance} = \frac{\text{driving pressure } (\Delta P)}{\text{flow}} \propto \frac{\text{viscosity } (\eta) \times \text{length}}{(\text{radius})^4}$$

Viscosity increases in:
1. Polycythemia
2. Hyperproteinemic states (e.g., multiple myeloma)
3. Hereditary spherocytosis

Viscosity depends mostly on hematocrit.

Capillary fluid exchange

Four forces known as Starling forces determine fluid movement through capillary membranes:

P_c = capillary pressure—tends to move fluid out of capillary

P_i = interstitial fluid pressure—tends to move fluid into capillary

π_c = plasma colloid osmotic pressure—tends to cause osmosis of fluid into capillary

π_i = interstitial fluid colloid osmotic pressure—tends to cause osmosis of fluid out of capillary

K_f = filtration constant

Thus net filtration pressure = $P_{net} = [(P_c - P_i) - (\pi_c - \pi_i)]K_f$

Cardiac cycle

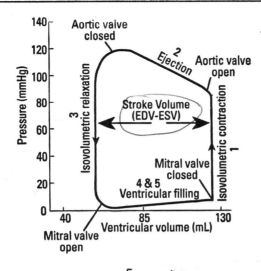

Phases:

1. Isovolumetric contraction—period between mitral valve closure and aortic valve opening; period of highest oxygen consumption
2. Systolic ejection—period between aortic valve opening and closing
3. Isovolumetric relaxation—period between aortic valve closing and mitral valve opening
4. Rapid filling—period just after mitral valve opening
5. Slow filling—period just before mitral valve closure

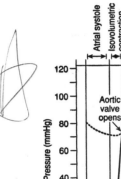

S1—mitral and tricuspid valve closure.
S2—aortic and pulmonary valveclosure.
S3—end of rapid ventricular filling.
S4—high atrial pressure/stiff ventricle.

S3 is associated with dilated CHF.
S4 is associated with hypertrophic CHF.

a wave: atrial contraction.
c wave: RV contraction (tricuspidvalve bulging into atrium).
v wave: ↑ atrial pressure due to filling against closed tricuspid valve.

A: **A**trial contraction.
C: RV **C**ontraction/**C**arotid pulse.
V: **V**enous return against closed **V**alve.

Physiology

HIGH-YIELD FACTS

Electrocardiogram

P wave—atrial depolarization.
P-R interval—conduction delay through AV node.
QRS complex—ventricular depolarization.
Q-T interval—mechanical contraction of the ventricles.
T wave—ventricular repolarization.
Atrial repolarization is masked by QRS complex.
Secondary or tertiary AV block means many P waves for each QRS.

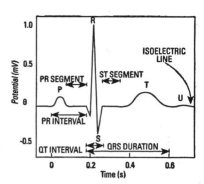

Arterial baroreceptors

Receptors:
1. Aortic arch transmits via vagus nerve to medulla
2. Carotid sinus transmits via glossopharyngeal nerve to medulla

↑ arterial pressure → ↑ stretch → ↑ afferent baroreceptor firing → ↓ sympathetic firing and ↑ efferent parasympathetic stimulation → vasodilation, ↓HR, ↓ contractility, ↓ BP.

Chemoreceptors

Peripheral

Central

1. Aortic bodies: respond to decreased Po_2, increased Pco_2 of blood
2. Carotid bodies: respond to decreased Po_2, increased Pco_2, and decreased pH of blood

Respond to changes in pH and Pco_2 of brain interstitial fluid, which in turn are influenced by arterial CO_2. Do not directly respond to Po_2.

Electrophysiological differences between skeletal and cardiac muscle

In contrast to skeletal muscle:
1. Cardiac muscle action potential has a plateau, which is due to Ca^{2+} influx
2. Cardiac nodal cells spontaneously depolarize, resulting in automaticity
3. Cardiac myocytes are electrically coupled to each other by gap junctions
4. Cardiac muscle contraction is dependent on extracellular calcium, which stimulates calcium release from the cardiac muscle sarcoplasmic reticulum (calcium-induced calcium release)

Fetal circulation

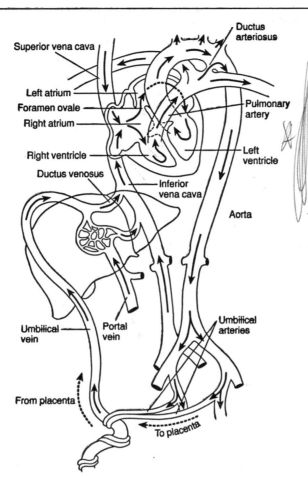

Superior vena cava

Left atrium

Foramen ovale

Right atrium

Right ventricle

Ductus venosus

Inferior vena cava

Ductus arteriosus

Pulmonary artery

Left ventricle

Aorta

Umbilical vein

Portal vein

Umbilical arteries

From placenta

To placenta

Blood in umbilical vein is ≈ 80% saturated with O_2.

Most oxygenated blood reaching the heart via IVC is diverted through the foramen ovale and pumped out the aorta to the head.

Deoxygenated blood from the SVC is expelled into the pulmonary artery and ductus arteriosus to the lower body of the fetus.

Control of mean arterial pressure

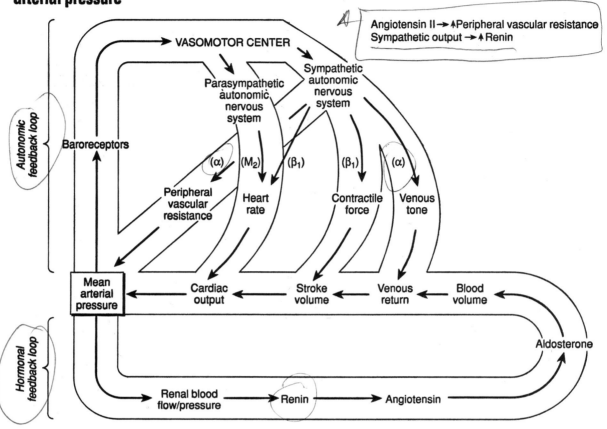

Angiotensin II → ↑Peripheral vascular resistance
Sympathetic output → ↑Renin

Circulation through organs

Liver: largest share of systemic cardiac output.
Kidney: highest blood flow per gram of tissue.
Heart: large arteriovenous O_2 difference. Increased O_2 demand is met by increased coronary blood flow, not by increased extraction of O_2.

Autoregulation

Sites: brain, kidney, heart
Mechanism: in the brain and heart, blood flow is altered to meet demands of tissue via local metabolites (e.g., nitric oxide). In the kidney, local metabolites maintain renal artery pressure constant.

The pulmonary vasculature is unique in that hypoxia causes vasoconstriction (in other organs hypoxia causes vasodilation).

Physiology

HIGH-YIELD FACTS

Response to high altitude

1. Acute increase in ventilation by 65%
2. Chronic increase in ventilation
3. ↑ erythropoietin → ↑ hematocrit and hemoglobin concentration
4. Increased 2,3-DPG (Hb releases O_2 more readily)
5. Cellular changes (increased mitochondria)
6. Increased renal excretion of bicarbonate to compensate for the respiratory alkalosis

---

Important lung products

1. **S**urfactant: ↓ alveolar surface tension
2. **P**rostaglandins
3. **H**istamine
4. **A**ngiotensin converting enzyme (ACE): AI → AII; inactivates bradykinin
5. **K**allikrein: activates bradykinin

Even the lungs get a big **SPHAK** attack!

Particle size and lung entrapment

Diameter of:

> 10 μm: Trapped by nostril hairs or settle on mucous membranes in nose and pharynx.

2–10 μm: Fall on bronchial walls → reflex bronchial constriction and coughing. Also removed by cilia.

0.5–2 μm: Reach alveoli → ingested by macrophages.

< 0.5 μm: Remain suspended in air.

Kartagener's syndrome = immotile cilia due to a dynein arm defect. Bacteria and particles not pushed out (also sperm cilia inactive). Results in bronchiectasis, situs inversus, sterility, and recurrent sinusitis.

Lung volumes

1. Residual volume (RV) = air in lung at maximal expiration
2. Expiratory reserve volume (ERV) = air that can still be breathed out after normal expiration
3. Tidal volume (TV) = air that moves into lung with each inspiration
4. Inspiratory reserve volume (IRV) = air in excess of tidal volume that moves into lung on maximum inspiration
5. Vital capacity = TV + IRV + ERV
6. Functional reserve capacity = RV + ERV
7. Inspiratory capacity = IRV + TV

Vital capacity is everything but the residual volume.

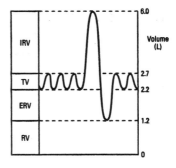

Physiology

HIGH-YIELD FACTS

Oxygen dissociation curve

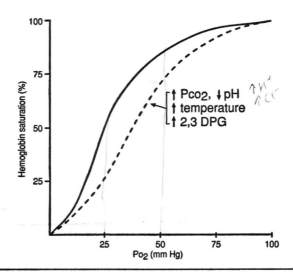

When curve shifts to the right, ↓ affinity of hemoglobin for O_2 (facilitates unloading of O_2 to tissue).

↑ Pco_2, ↓ pH
↑ temperature
↑ 2,3 DPG

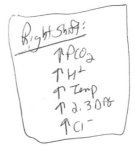

[handwritten: Right Shift: ↑PCO₂, ↑H⁺, ↑Temp, ↑2,3DPG, ↑Cl⁻]

Acid-base physiology

	pH	Pco_2	[HCO_3^-]	Cause	Compensatory response
Met. acidosis	↓	↓	↓	Diabetic ketoacidosis; diarrhea	Hyperventilation
Resp. acidosis	↓	↑	↑	COPD; airway obstruction	Renal [HCO_3^-] reabsorption
Resp. alkalosis	↑	↓	↓	High altitude	Renal [HCO_3^-] secretion
Met. alkalosis	↑	↑	↑	Vomiting	Hypoventilation

Pulmonary circulation

Normally a low-resistance, high-compliance system keeps pulmonary blood pressure low. With increased Pco_2 (e.g., exercise), a low pulmonary blood pressure is maintained by vasodilating normally closed apical capillaries, thereby lowering pulmonary resistance.

A consequence of primary pulmonary hypertension is cor pulmonale and subsequent right ventricular failure.

V/Q mismatch

Ideally, ventilation is matched to perfusion (i.e., V/Q = 1) in order for adequate oxygenation to occur efficiently.

Lung zones:
Apex of the lung: V/Q = 3 (wasted ventilation)
Base of the lung: V/Q = 0.6 (wasted perfusion)
Both ventilation and perfusion are greater at the base of the lung than at the apex of the lung.

With exercise (increased cardiac output), there is vasodilation of apical capillaries, resulting in a V/Q ratio that approaches unity. Certain organisms that thrive in high O_2 (e.g., TB) flourish in the apex.

CO₂ transport

Carbon dioxide is transported from tissues to the lungs in 3 forms:

1. Bicarbonate (65%)

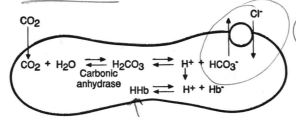

Deoxyhemoglobin binds H⁺ more actively than does oxyhemoglobin (Bohr effect).

2. Bound to hemoglobin as carbaminohemoglobin (25%)
3. Dissolved CO_2 (10%)

Obstructive lung disease

Obstruction of air flow, resulting in air trapping in the lungs. Pulmonary function tests: decreased FEV_1/FVC ratio (hallmark).

Types:

1. Bronchiectasis—chronic necrotizing infection of bronchi → dilated airways, purulent sputum, recurrent infections, hemoptysis. Associated with bronchial obstruction, cystic fibrosis, poor ciliary motility.
2. Chronic bronchitis ("blue bloaters")—sputum production for greater than 3 consecutive months in two or more years. Reid index > 50% (hypertrophy of mucus-secreting glands in the bronchioles).
3. Emphysema ("pink puffer")—enlargement of airspaces and decreased recoil resulting from destruction of alveolar walls. Caused by smoking (centroacinar emphysema) and α_1-antitrypsin deficiency (panacinar emphysema and liver cirrhosis) → ↑ elastase activity.
4. Asthma—airway hyperresponsiveness causes reversible bronchoconstriction. Can be triggered by viral URIs, allergens, and stress.

Restrictive lung disease

Decreased lung volumes (decreased VC and TLC).

Types:

1. Poor breathing mechanics (extrapulmonary):
   a. Poor muscular effort: polio, myasthenia gravis.
   b. Poor apparatus: scoliosis.
2. Poor lung expansion (pulmonary):
   a. Defective alveolar filling: pneumonia, ARDS.
   b. Interstitial fibrosis: causes increased recoil, thereby limiting alveolar expansion. PFTs reveal an FEV_1/FVC ratio > 90%. Complications include cor pulmonale. Can be seen in diffuse interstitial pulmonary fibrosis and bleomycin toxicity.

PHYSIOLOGY—GASTROINTESTINAL

Pancreatic exocrine secretion

Secretory acini synthesize and secrete zymogens, stimulated by acetylcholine and CCK. Pancreatic ducts secrete mucus and alkaline fluid when stimulated by secretin.

Pancreatic enzymes	Alpha-amylase: starch digestion, secreted in active form.
	Lipase, phospholipase A, colipase: fat digestion.
	Proteases (trypsin, chymotrypsin, elastase, carboxypeptidases): protein digestion, secreted as proenzymes.
	Trypsinogen is converted to active enzyme trypsin by enteropeptidase, a duodenal brush-border enzyme. Trypsin then activates the other proenzymes and can also activate trypsinogen (positive-feedback loop).

Stimulation of pancreatic functions

Secretin	Stimulates flow of bicarbonate-containing fluid.
Cholecystokinin	Major stimulus for zymogen release, weak stimulus for alkaline fluid flow.
Acetylcholine	Major stimulus for zymogen release, poor stimulus for bicarbonate secretion.
Somatostatin	Inhibits the release of gastrin and secretin.

Bilirubin	Product of heme metabolism, actively taken up by hepatocytes. Conjugated version is water soluble.

Bile	Secreted by hepatocytes. Composed of bile salts, phospholipids, cholesterol, bilirubin, water (97%). Bile salts are amphipathic (hydrophilic and hydrophobic domains) and solubilize lipids in micelles for absorption.

Carbohydrate digestion

Only monosaccharides are absorbed.

Salivary amylase	Starts digestion, hydrolyzes alpha-1,4 linkages to give maltose, maltotriose, and dextrans.
Pancreatic amylase	Highest concentration in duodenal lumen, hydrolyzes starch to oligosaccharides, maltose, and maltotriose.
Oligosaccharide hydrolases	At brush border of intestine, is the rate-limiting step in carbohydrate digestion, produces monosaccharides.

Salivary secretion

Source	Parotid, submandibular, and sublingual glands.	Salivary secretion is stimulated by both sympathetic and parasympathetic activity.
Function	1. Alpha-amylase (ptyalin) begins starch digestion	
	2. Neutralizes oral bacterial acids, maintains dental health	
	3. Mucins (glycoproteins) lubricate food	

Glucose absorption	Occurs at duodenum and proximal jejunum.
	Absorbed across cell membrane by sodium-glucose-coupled transporter.

Stomach secretions

	Purpose	Source
Mucus	Lubricant, protects surface from H^+	Mucous cell
Intrinsic factor	Vitamin B_{12} absorption (in small intestine)	Parietal cell
H^+	Kills bacteria, breaks down food, converts pepsinogen	Parietal cell
Pepsinogen	Broken down to pepsin (a protease)	Chief cell
Gastrin	Stimulates acid secretion	G cell

GI secretory products

	Source	Function	Regulation	Notes
Intrinsic factor	Parietal cells (stomach)	Vitamin B_{12} binding protein required for vitamin's uptake in terminal ileum		Autoimmune destruction of parietal cells → chronic gastritis → pernicious anemia
Gastric acid	Parietal cells	Lowers pH to optimal range for pepsin function. Sterilizes chyme	Stimulated by histamine, ACh, gastrin. Inhibited by prostaglandin	Not essential for digestion. Inadequate acid → ↑ risk *Salmonella* infections
Pepsin	Chief cells (stomach)	Begins protein digestion; optimal function at pH 1.0–3.0	Stimulated by vagal input, local acid	Inactive pepsinogen converted to pepsin by H^+
Gastrin	G cells of antrum and duodenum	1. Stimulates secretion of HCl, IF and pepsinogen 2. Stimulates gastric motility	Stimulated by stomach distention, amino acids, peptides, vagus (via GRP); inhibited by secretin and stomach acid pH < 1.5	Hypersecreted in Zollinger–Ellison syndrome → peptic ulcers. Phenylalanine and tryptophan are most potent stimulators.
Bicarbonate	Surface submucosal cells of stomach and duodenum	Neutralizes acid: forms an unstirred layer with mucus on luminal surface, preventing autodigestion		
Cholecystokinin (CCK)	I cells of duodenum and jejunum.	1. Stimulates gallbladder contraction 2. Stimulates pancreatic enzyme secretion 3. Inhibits gastric emptying	Stimulated by fatty acids, amino acids	In cholelithiasis, pain worsens after eating fatty foods due to CCK release → gallbladder contraction
Secretin	S cells of duodenum	Nature's antacid: 1. Stimulates pancreatic HCO_3^- secretion 2. Inhibits gastric acid secretion	Stimulated by acid and fatty acids in lumen of duodenum	Alkaline pancreatic juice in duodenum neutralizes gastric acid, allowing pancreatic enzymes to function
Somatostatin	D cells in pancreatic islets, gastrointestinal mucosa	Inhibits: 1. Gastric acid and pepsinogen secretion 2. Pancreatic and small intestine fluid secretion 3. Gallbladder contraction 4. Release of both insulin and glucagon	Stimulated by acid; inhibited by vagus	Very inhibitory hormone; anti-growth hormone effects (↓ digestion and ↓ absorption of substances needed for growth)

Regulation of gastric acid secretion

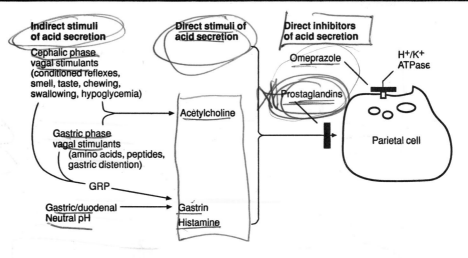

Indirect stimuli of acid secretion

Cephalic phase vagal stimulants (conditioned reflexes, smell, taste, chewing, swallowing, hypoglycemia)

Gastric phase vagal stimulants (amino acids, peptides, gastric distention)

GRP

Gastric/duodenal Neutral pH

Direct stimuli of acid secretion

Acetylcholine

Gastrin

Histamine

Direct inhibitors of acid secretion

Omeprazole

Prostaglandins

H^+/K^+ ATPase

Parietal cell

PHYSIOLOGY—RENAL

Filtration fraction

$$FF = GFR/RPF$$
$$GFR = C_{inulin} \approx C_{creatinine}$$
$$RPF = C_{PAH}$$

Renal clearance

$C_x = U \times V / P_x$ = volume of plasma from which the substance is cleared completely per unit time.

If $C_x <$ GFR, then there is net tubular reabsorption of X.

If $C_x >$ GFR, then there is net tubular secretion of X.

If $C_x =$ GFR, then no net secretion or reabsorption.

Glomerular filtration rate

$$GFR = U_{Inulin} \times V / P_{Inulin} = C_{Inulin}$$

Inulin is freely filtered and is neither reabsorbed nor secreted.

Effective renal plasma flow

$$ERPF = U_{PAH} \times V / P_{PAH} = C_{PAH} = RBF (1 - Hct)$$

PAH is filtered and secreted.

PAH

Secreted in proximal tubule.

Active transport process, requires ATP, inhibited by cyanide.

Mediated by a carrier system for organic acids, competitively inhibited by probenecid.

Glucose clearance

Glucose at normal level is completely reabsorbed (99% in proximal tubule, 1% in collecting ducts). Mechanism is saturable.

reabsorbed in prox tubule

Symport

Renal threshold is 200 mg/dl of arterial plasma.

Amino acids clearance

Reabsorption by at least 3 distinct carrier systems, with competitive inhibition within each group. Active transport occurs in proximal tubule and is saturable.

reabsorbed in prox tubule

Electrolyte clearance

Sodium	>99% of filtered load is absorbed. Reabsorption is active throughout most of nephron.
Chloride	Reabsorption is passive, driven by electrochemical gradients maintained by sodium reabsorption (except at thick ascending loop of Henle).

Measuring fluid compartments

Compartment	Direct measurement
Total body water (TBW)	Antipyrine, tritium
Extracellular fluid (⅓ TBW)	Inulin, mannitol
Plasma	Evans blue, I^{131}-albumin

	Indirect measurement
Interstitial fluid	Extracellular fluid – plasma
Intracellular fluid (⅔ TBW)	TBW – extracellular fluid

Kidney endocrine functions

Endocrine functions of the kidney:

1. Endothelial cells of peritubular capillaries secrete erythropoietin in response to hypoxia
2. Conversion of 25-OH vit. D to 1,25-$(OH)_2$ vit. D by 1α-hydroxylase, which is activated by PTH
3. JG cells secrete renin in response to ↓ renal arterial pressure and ↑ renal nerve discharge
4. Secretion of prostaglandins that vasodilate the afferent arteriole to increase GFR

NSAIDs can cause renal failure by inhibiting the renal production of prostaglandins, which keep the afferent arteriole vasodilated to maintain GFR.

Glomerular filtration barrier

Composed of:

1. Fenestrated capillary endothelium (size barrier)
2. Fused basement membrane with heparan sulfate (negative charge barrier)
3. Epithelial layer consisting of podocyte foot processes

The charge barrier is lost in nephrotic syndrome, resulting in albuminuria, hypoproteinemia, generalized edema, and hyperlipidemia.

Renal failure

Failure to make urine and excrete nitrogenous wastes. Consequences:

1. Anemia (failure of erythropoietin production)
2. Renal osteodystrophy (failure of active vit. D production)
3. Hyperkalemia, which can lead to cardiac arrhythmias
4. Metabolic acidosis due to ↓ acid excretion and ↓ generation of buffers
5. Uremia (increased BUN/creatinine)
6. Sodium and H_2O excess → CHF and pulmonary edema

Two forms of renal failure: Acute renal failure (often due to hypoxia) and chronic renal failure.

Hormones acting on kidney

	Stimulus for secretion	Action on kidneys
Vasopressin (ADH)	↑ plasma osmolarity ↓ blood volume	↑ H₂O permeability of principal cells in collecting ducts
Aldosterone	↓ blood volume (via AII) ↑ plasma [K⁺]	↑ Na⁺ reabsorption, ↑ K⁺ secretion, ↑ H⁺ secretion in distal tubule
Angiotensin II	↓ blood volume (via renin)	Contraction of mesangial cells → ↓ GFR ↑ Na⁺ and HCO₃⁻ reabsorption in proximal tubule
Atrial natriuretic peptide (ANP)	↑ atrial pressure	↓ Na⁺ reabsorption ↑ GFR
PTH	↓ plasma [Ca²⁺]	↑ Ca²⁺ reabsorption, ↓ PO₄³⁻ reabsorption, ↑ 1,25 (OH)₂ vitamin D production

Renin-angiotensin system

Mechanism: renin is released by the kidneys upon sensing ↓ BP and serves to cleave angiotensinogen to angiotensin I (AI) (a decapeptide). AI is then cleaved by angiotensin-converting enzyme (ACE) in the lung capillaries to angiotensin II (an octapeptide). Actions:

1. Potent vasoconstriction
2. Release of aldosterone from the adrenal cortex
3. Release of ADH from posterior pituitary
4. Stimulates hypothalamus → ↑ thirst

Overall, AII serves to ↑ intravascular volume and ↑ BP.

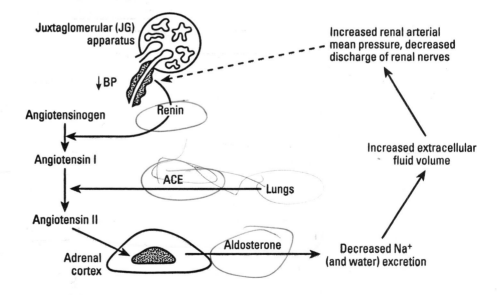

Hyperaldosteronism

Primary hyperaldosteronism (Conn's syndrome). Caused by an aldosterone-secreting tumor, resulting in hypertension, hypokalemia, hypernatremia, metabolic alkalosis, and low plasma renin. Secondary hyperaldosteronism. Due to renal artery stenosis and chronic renal failure (CHF, cirrhosis, nephrotic). Kidney misperception of low intravascular volume, resulting in an overactive renin-angiotensin system. Therefore, it is associated with high plasma renin.

Treatment includes spironolactone, a diuretic that works by acting as an aldosterone antagonist.

Nephron physiology

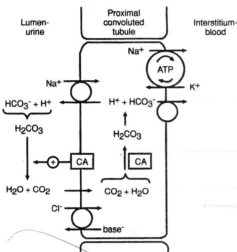

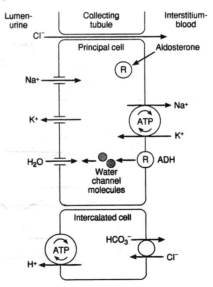

- Thin descending loop of Henle—passively reabsorbs water via medullar hypertonicity (impermeable to sodium).
- Thick ascending loop of Henle—actively reabsorbs Na^+, K^+, Cl^- and indirectly induces the reabsorption of Mg^{2+} and Ca^{2+}.

- Proximal convoluted tubule—"workhorse of the nephron." Reabsorbs all of the glucose and amino acids and most of the bicarbonate, sodium, and water. Secretes ammonia, which acts as a buffer for secreted H^+.

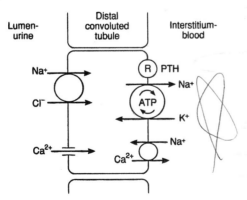

- Distal convoluted tubule—actively reabsorbs Na^+, Cl^-. Reabsorption of Ca^{2+} is under the control of PTH.

- Collecting tubules—reabsorb Na^+ in exchange for secreting K^+ or H^+ (regulated by aldosterone). Reabsorption of water is regulated by ADH.

Physiology

HIGH-YIELD FACTS

Steroid/thyroid hormone mechanism

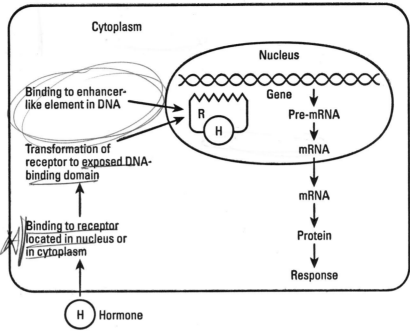

Cytoplasm

Nucleus

Binding to enhancer-like element in DNA

R

H

Gene

Pre-mRNA

mRNA

Transformation of receptor to exposed DNA-binding domain

mRNA

Binding to receptor located in nucleus or in cytoplasm

Protein

Response

(H) Hormone

Insulin-independent organs

Muscle and adipose tissue depend on insulin for glucose uptake. Brain and RBCs take up glucose independent of insulin levels.

Brain and RBCs depend on glucose for metabolism under normal circumstances.

Pituitary glycoprotein hormones

Pituitary glycoprotein hormones are TSH, LH, FSH.
α subunit – common subunit to TSH, LH, FSH and hCG.
β subunit – determines hormone specificity.

T.S.H. and **TSH** = The Sex Hormones and **TSH**

PTH

Source Chief cells of parathyroid.

Function
1. Increase bone resorption of calcium + phosphate
2. Increase kidney reabsorption of calcium
3. Decrease kidney reabsorption of phosphate
4. Increase 1,25 (OH)$_2$ vit. D production (cholecalciferol) by stimulating kidney 1α-hydroxylase

PTH: increases serum Ca^{2+}, decreases serum PO_4^{3-}, increases urine PO_4^{3-}.
PTH stimulates both osteoclasts and osteoblasts.

Regulation Increases in serum Ca^{2+} decrease secretion.

Calcitonin

Source Parafollicular cells (C cells) of thyroid.

Function
1. Decrease bone resorption of calcium
2. Increase urinary excretion of calcium

Calcitonin rhymes with "bone in."
Calcitonin opposes actions of PTH and acts faster than PTH. It's probably not important in normal calcium homeostasis.

Regulation Increases in serum Ca^{2+} increase secretion.

Vitamin D

Source	Vitamin D_3 from sun exposure in skin. D_2 from plants. Both converted to 25-OH vit. D in liver and to 1,25-$(OH)_2$ vit. D in kidney.
Function	1. Increase absorption of dietary calcium 2. Increase absorption of dietary phosphate 3. Increase bone resorption of Ca^{2+} and PO_4^{3-}
Regulation	Increased PTH causes increased 1,25-(OH_2) vit. D conversion. Decreased phosphate causes increased 1,25-$(OH)_2$ vit. D conversion. 1,25-$(OH)_2$ vit. D feedback inhibits its own production.

If you don't get vit. D, you get rickets (kids) or osteomalacia (adults).

24,25-$(OH)_2$ vit. D is the inactive form of vit. D.

Estrogen

Source	Ovary (estradiol), placenta (estriol), blood (aromatization), testes.
Function	1. Growth of follicle 2. Endometrial proliferation, myometrial excitability 3. Genitalia development 4. Stromal development of breast 5. Fat deposition 6. Libido 7. Hepatic synthesis of transport proteins 8. Feedback inhibition of FSH 9. LH surge

Potency: estradiol > estrone > estriol

Menstrual cycle

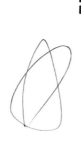
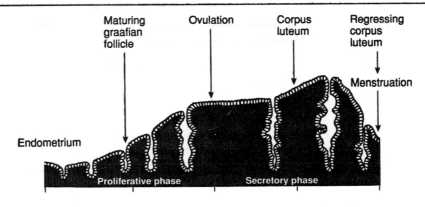
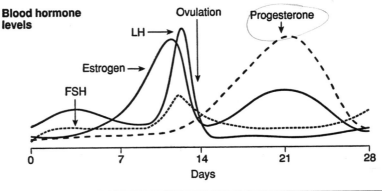
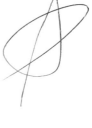

Physiology

HIGH-YIELD FACTS

Progesterone

Source	Corpus luteum, placenta, adrenal cortex, testes.
Function	1. Stimulation of endometrial glandular secretions and spiral artery development
	2. Maintenance of pregnancy
	3. Decreased myometrial excitability
	4. Production of thick cervical mucus, which inhibits sperm entry into the uterus
	5. Increased temperature (0.5 degree)
	6. Inhibition of gonadotropins (LH, FSH)
	7. Uterine smooth muscle relaxation

hCG

Source	Trophoblast, placenta
Function	1. Maintains the corpus luteum for the 1st trimester because it acts like LH but is not susceptible to feedback regulation from estrogen and progesterone. In the 2nd and 3rd trimester, the placenta synthesizes its own estrogen and progesterone. As a result, the corpus luteum degenerates.
	2. Used to detect pregnancy because it appears in the urine 8 days after successful fertilization.

Norepinephrine vs. epinephrine

	Epinephrine	Norepinephrine	
Receptor predominance	β > α	α ≫ β	Adrenal medullary cells and some neurons contain the enzyme PMNT, which converts norepinephrine to epinephrine.
Total peripheral resistance	↓	↑	
Cardiac output	↑	↓	
Heart rate	↑	↓ (reflex)	
Blood pressure	↑ pulse pressure	↑	

Male spermatogenesis

Pituitary	Testes	Products	Functions of products

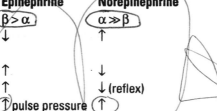

FSH ⟶ Sertoli cell ⟶ Androgen binding protein — Ensures that testosterone in seminiferous tubule is high

Inhibin — Inhibits FSH

LH ⟶ Leydig cell ⟶ Testosterone — Differentiates male genitalia, has anabolic effects on protein metabolism, maintains gametogenesis, maintains libido, inhibits LH, and fuses epiphyseal plates in bone

FSH → Sertoli cells → Sperm production
LH → Leydig cells

Cardiovascular
1. Basic electrocardiographic changes (e.g., Q waves, ST segment).
2. Effects of electrolyte abnormalities on the heart (e.g., potassium and calcium)
3. Physiologic effects of the Valsalva maneuver.
4. Blood gas physiology at high altitude.

Endocrine/Reproductive
1. Physiologic features of hyperparathyroidism and associated laboratory findings.
2. Clinical tests for endocrine abnormalities (e.g., glucose tolerance, dexamethasone suppression).
3. Diseases associated with hormonal abnormalities (e.g., Cushing's disease, diabetes insipidus).
4. Sites of hormone production during pregnancy (e.g., corpus luteum, placenta).
5. Regulation of prolactin secretion.
6. Hormonal changes and physiologic effects associated with menopause.

Gastrointestinal
1. Sites of absorption of major nutrients (e.g., ileum: vit. B_{12}).
2. Bile production and enterohepatic circulation.
3. Glucose cotransport into cells of gut and peripheral tissues.

Pulmonary
1. Calculation of alveolar oxygen tension (i.e., alveolar air equation) and alveolar to arterial oxygen gradient.
2. Mechanical differences between inspiration and expiration.
3. Characteristic pulmonary function curves for common lung diseases (e.g., bronchitis, emphysema, asthma, interstitial lung disease).
4. Gas diffusion across alveolocapillary membrane.

Renal/Acid-Base
1. Differences among active transport, facilitated diffusion, and diffusion.
2. Distinguishing differences between central and nephrogenic diabetes insipidus.

General
1. Role of calmodulin and troponin C in muscle activation.
2. Role of ions (e.g., calcium, sodium, magnesium, potassium) in cardiac and muscle cells.
3. The clotting cascade and clotting factors which require vitamin K for synthesis (II, VII, IX, X).

HIGH-YIELD FACTS

Physiology

Database of Basic Science Review Resources

Comprehensive
Anatomy
Behavioral Science
Biochemistry
Microbiology
Pathology
Pharmacology
Physiology
Commercial Review Courses
Publisher Contacts

This section is a database of current basic science review books, sample examination books and commercial review courses marketed to medical students studying for the USMLE Step 1. At the end of this section is a list of publishers and independent bookstores with addresses and phone numbers. For each book, we list the **Title** of the book, the **First Author** (or editor), the **Series Name** (where applicable), the **Current Publisher,** the **Copyright Year,** the **Number of Pages,** the **ISBN Code,** the **Approximate List Price,** the **Format** of the book, and the **Number of Test Questions.** The entries for most books also include **Summary Comments** that describe their style and overall utility for studying. Finally, each book receives a **Rating.** The books are sorted into a comprehensive section as well as into sections corresponding to the seven traditional basic medical science disciplines (anatomy, behavioral science, biochemistry, microbiology, pathology, pharmacology, and physiology). Within each section they are sorted first by Rating, then by Title, and lastly by Author.

For the 1996 edition of *First Aid for the USMLE Step 1,* the database of review books has been expanded and updated, with over 30 new books and software and more in-depth summary comments. A letter rating scale with ten different grades reflects the detailed student evaluations. Each book receives a rating as follows:

A+	Excellent for boards review.
A A–	Very good for boards review; choose among the group.
B+ B B–	Good, but use only after exhausting better sources.
C+ C C–	Fair, but many better books in the discipline, or low-yield subject material.
D	Not appropriate.

The **Rating** is meant to reflect the overall usefulness of the book in preparing for the USMLE Step 1 examination. This is based on a number of factors, including:

- The cost of the book.
- The readability of the text.
- The appropriateness and accuracy of the book.
- The quality and number of sample questions.
- The quality of written answers to sample questions.
- The quality and utility of visual aids (i.e., graphs, diagrams, photographs, etc.).
- The length of the text (longer is not necessarily better).
- The quality and number of other books available in the same discipline.
- The importance of the discipline on the USMLE Step 1 examination.

Please note that the rating does **not** reflect the quality of the book for purposes other than reviewing for the USMLE Step 1 examination. Many books with low ratings are well written and informative, but are not ideal for boards preparation. We have also avoided listing or commenting on the wide variety of general textbooks available in the basic sciences.

The evaluations are based on formal and informal surveys of thousands of medical students at many medical schools across the country. The summary comments and overall ratings represent a consensus opinion, but there may have been a large range of opinion or limited student feedback on one particular book.

Please note that the data listed are subject to change:

- Publishers' prices change frequently.
- Individual bookstores often charge an additional markup.
- New editions come out frequently, and the quality of updating varies.
- The same book may be reissued through another publisher.

We actively encourage medical students and faculty to submit their opinions and ratings of these basic science review books so that we may update our database. (*See* How to Contribute, page xv.) In addition, we ask that publishers and authors submit review copies of basic science review books, including new editions and books not included in our database for evaluation. We also solicit reviews of new books or suggestions for alternate modes of study that may be useful in preparing for the examination, such as flashcards, computer-based tutorials, and commercial review courses.

Disclaimer

No material in this book, including the ratings, reflects the opinion or influence of the publisher. All errors and omissions will gladly be corrected if brought to the attention of the authors through the publisher. Please note that the book *Underground Guide to Retired and Self-Test Questions* (p. 221) is an independent publication by the authors of this book; its rating is based solely on data from the student survey.

Retired NBME Basic Medical Sciences Test Items
— Test/993 q

NBME

NBME, 1991, 136 pages, Out of print

Contains "retired" questions in all seven areas of basic science. Excellent topics. Letter answers only with no explanations. Content still relevant, although format outdated. No clinical vignettes. High yield. Out of print. Try to find an old copy. Not available in bookstores. Explanatory answers available in a separate publication (*Underground Guide,* see below).

Review for USMLE Step 1 Examination
$35.00 Test/1000+ q

NMS, Lazo

Williams & Wilkins, 1994, 331 pages, ISBN 0683062654

Very good source of practice questions and answers. Features updated clinical questions and vignettes. Some questions too picky or difficult. Good buy for the number of questions. Organized as four 200-question booklets; good for simulating the exam.

Self-Test in the Part I Basic Medical Sciences
— Test/630 q

NBME

NBME, 1989, 91 pages, Out of print

A very good source of questions, level of difficulty, and detail, although format very outdated. Ninety items per discipline. Letter answers with no explanations. No clinical vignettes. Out of print. Try to find an old copy. Not available in bookstores. Explanatory answers available in a separate publication (*Underground Guide,* see below).

Appleton & Lange's Review for the USMLE Step I
$34.95 Test/1200 q

Barton

Appleton & Lange, 1993, 263 pages, ISBN 0838502253

Good questions with very good answers. Many questions very picky. Questions organized by subject and indexed by subtopic. Good buy for the number of questions. Few clinical vignettes. A very good, straightforward, question-based review to assess your strengths and weaknesses. Weak anatomy section. New edition with revised anatomy section expected in early 1996.

Underground Guide to Retired and Self-Test Questions
$19.95 Review

Amin

S_2S Medical, 1996, 387 pages

Concise explanation guide to 1600+ *NBME Retired* and *Self-Test* questions. Easy read. Useful with or without NBME questions (not included). Referenced to current textbooks. First edition contained some incomplete explanations and errors. New edition features expanded and updated explanations. Not available in bookstores. Can be ordered at (800) 247-6553 or by fax at (419) 281-6883; fully refundable.

B MEPC USMLE Step 1 Review

$29.95   Test/1200 q

Fayemi
Appleton & Lange, 1996, 455 pages, ISBN 0838562698
New edition features questions with revised explanatory answers. Mixed-quality questions. Includes new clinical vignettes.

B Preparation for USMLE Step 1 Basic Medical Sciences, Volumes A, B, C

$14.00 ea   Test/315 q

Luder
Maval Medical Education, 1995, 70 pages, ISBN 1884083099 (Vol. A), 1884083202 (Vol. B), 1884083010 (Vol. C)
Well-written style questions with explanatory answers. Recently revised. Good color photographs. Many typographic errors and expensive for the number of questions.

B⁻ Preparation for the USMLE Step 1 Basic Medical Sciences, Volumes D, E

$14.00 ea   Test/210 q

Luder
Maval Medical Education, 1995, 54 pages, ISBN 1884083129
Same format and comments as for Volumes A, B, C but even more expensive for the number of questions.

B⁻ Rypin's Questions and Answers for Basic Science Review, Vol. II

$29.95   Test/1640 q

Frolich
Lippincott, 1993, 211 pages, ISBN 0397512473
Questions with detailed answers to supplement *Rypin's Medical Boards Review.* Decent overall question-based review of all subjects. Not referenced to a text. Requires time commitment.

C⁺ Basic Science

$75.00   Test/3500 q

FMSG
FMSG, 301 pages
Advertised as questions "remembered" from past NBME exams. Variable-quality questions with letter answers only. Poor photo quality. Contains outdated K-type and C-type (A/B/both/neither) items. Not available in bookstores. Can be ordered at (800) 662-3244, nonrefundable.

Basic Science Update 1993

$25.00   Test/332 q

FMSG

FMSG, 1993, 46 pages

An addendum to FMSG's *Basic Science*. Mixed-quality questions with letter answers only. Includes extended matching questions. Expensive. Can
be ordered at (800) 662-3244, non-refundable. Separate updates based on
recent USMLE administrations.

Basic Science Update 1994

$50.00   Test/727 q

FMSG

FMSG, 1994, 124 pages

Limited student feedback. Second in a series of FMSG. Also poor buy for
number of questions. Can be ordered at (800) 662-3244, non-refundable.

Clinical Anatomy and Pathophysiology for the Health Professional

$17.95   Review only

Stewart

MedMaster, 1994, 260 pages, ISBN 0940780062

Written for non-MD professionals. Not boards oriented. Simplistic, but may
be a good place to start for some students. Good diagrams.

Future Test: USMLE Step 1

$49.95   Software

National Learning Corp.

Future Technologies, 1994, ISBN 0837394538

PC software features multiple ways to review and self-test from database
of questions with explanations. Question styles not representative of current exam. Few clinical vignettes.

Medical Student's Guide to Top Board Scores

$15.95   Review

Rogers

Little, Brown, 1995, ISBN 0316754366

Old edition, easy to read, but information is low yield and coverage of topics is spotty. Contains some good mnemonics in basic and clinical sciences, but not necessarily boards-relevant. Incomplete and very outdated
list of recommended books for board review. New edition not yet reviewed.

PASS USMLE Step 1: Practice by Assessing Study Skills

$19.95   How-to/500 q

Schwenker

Little, Brown, 1995, 140 pages, ISBN 0316776009

Detailed review of study and testing strategies for standardized exams and
medical school. Worth considering if you have study or testing difficulties.
Includes diagnostic test.

REVIEW RESOURCES

Comprehensive

REVIEW RESOURCES

Comprehensive

Rypin's Basic Sciences Review, Vol. I
Frohlich

$34.95   Review/1000+ q

Lippincott, 1993, 856 pages, ISBN 0397512457
Multi-topic textbook with very few figures and tables. A good general reference, but should be used with other subject-specific sources. Well-priced for the number of pages and questions. Requires extensive time commitment.

Study Skills and Test-Taking Strategies for Medical Students
Oklahoma Notes, Shain

$17.95   How-to only

Springer-Verlag, 1995, 204 pages, ISBN 038794396X
Very detailed discussion of study skills for medical school. May be useful for some students seeking a structured approach, but probably not necessary for most medical students.

The Most Common Manual for Medical Students
Grosso

$14.95   Review only

Stephen Grosso, 1991, 487 pages, ISBN 0963335405
A compilation of over 3500 "most common questions" of medicine. Well organized, compact. Useful for the wards, with some high-yield basic science material mixed in with the clinical material.

Year Book's Medical Licensure Review: Basic Sciences
Bollet

$45.95   Review/250 q

Mosby-Year Book, 1989, 510 pages, ISBN 0815110219
Detailed textbook approach to all subjects. Questions with letter answers only. Some good illustrations. Clinically correlated. Text needs updating. Worth considering, but requires time commitment.

How to Prepare for the USMLE Step 1
Thornborough

$14.95   How-to/400 q

McGraw-Hill, 1993, 216 pages, ISBN 0070645221
A detailed but not very useful "how-to-prepare" book written for the new examination. Uses questions from other PreTest books. Sixteen 25-question practice tests divided by topic. Contains an alphabetical list of 2000 medical terms of dubious value.

New Rudman's Questions and Answers on the USMLE $49.95 Test/280 q
Rudman
National Learning Corporation, 1991, 200 pages, ISBN 0837358043
Combines Step 1 and Step 2 questions but no explanations. Lacks references. Very expensive. Limited review of anatomy and physiology at the end of the book. Revised for the USMLE. Use only if other sources are exhausted.

PreTest Step 1 Simulated Exam $30.00 Test/420 q
Thornborough
McGraw-Hill, 1991, 64 pages, ISBN 0079110088
Typical PreTest questions, some repeated from PreTest book series. Letter answers only. Free computerized evaluation takes a long time to receive back from PreTest Center. New edition expected in 1995.

NEW BOOKS—COMPREHENSIVE

Basic Science Update 1995 — Test
FMSG
FMSG, 1995
Not yet reviewed. Most recent update to FMSG's *Basic Science* series.

Electronic Review for USMLE Step 1 $34.95 Software/1000+ q
NMS, Lazo
Williams & Wilkins, 1995, ISBN 0683062654
Not yet reviewed. For Windows, PC and Mac. Features same questions from NMS *Review for USMLE Step 1 Examination*. Has five simulation tests with user-friendly graphical interface. Provides detailed analysis of test performance. Also allows review of questions by subject. Copy protection mechanism is inconvenient.

Medical Boards–Step 1 Made Ridiculously Simple $21.95 Review
Carl
MedMaster, 1996, 260 pages, ISBN 0940780259
Expected in early 1996. Comprehensive review of basic sciences in chart form.

Mosby's USMLE Step 1 Exam: Basic Sciences $37.95 Review
Mosby
Mosby-Year Book, 1996, ISBN 0815169043
Expected in early 1996. Contains questions for self testing in both text and software format. Both Windows and Mac versions are planned. Money-back guarantee.

REVIEW RESOURCES

Comprehensive

Step 1 Success

$34.00   Test

Zaslau

FMSG, 1996, ISBN 1886468079

Expected in early 1996. Features full-length diagnostic test.

USMLE Success

$30.00   How-to/540 q.

Zaslau

FMSG, 1995, 170 pages, ISBN 1886468036

Not yet reviewed. Contains broad exam preparation advice and mnemonics for all three steps. Oriented towards international medical graduates. Questions with letter answers only.

Anatomy: Review for New National Boards
Johnson

$25.00   Test/506 q

J & S, 1992, 217 pages, ISBN 0963287303

Easy reading. Questions with detailed explanations. Good, superficial overview of cell biology, histology, gross anatomy, embryology, and neuroanatomy. Discusses clnically relevant anatomic science with adequate explanations, illustrations, and pictures and also many clinically relevant genetic diseases. Several key topics not covered. Includes good photomicrographs and cross-sectional imaging-based questions.

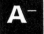

Clinical Neuroanatomy Made Ridiculously Simple
Goldberg

$11.95   Review/Few q

MedMaster, 1995, 89 pages, ISBN 0940780003

Easy to read, memorable, simplified, with clever diagrams. Very quick, high-yield review of neuroanatomy. Good emphasis on clinically relevant pathways, cranial nerves, and neurological diseases. Spotty coverage of some topics. Non-board-style questions.

High-Yield Neuroanatomy
Fix

$14.95   Review only

Williams & Wilkins, 1994, 111 pages, ISBN 0683032488

Clean outline format, easy to read. Straight forward text with excellent diagrams and illustrations. Some mislabeled diagrams. High-yield review in less than a day. Compare with *Clinical Neuroanatomy Made Ridiculously Simple.*

Clinical Anatomy Made Ridiculously Simple
Goldberg

$17.95   Review only

MedMaster, 1991, 175 pages, ISBN 094078002X

Easy reading, simple diagrams, lots of mnemonics, and "ridiculous" associations. Somewhat incomplete. This style does not appeal to all students, so browse before buying. Good review for the relatively low-yield subject of gross anatomy.

MEPC Anatomy
Wilson

$16.95   Test/700 q

Appleton & Lange, 1995, 251 pages, ISBN 0838562183

Updated with many clinical vignettes followed by questions. Includes gross anatomy, neuroanatomy, cell biology, embryology. Worth considering as alternative to J&S *Anatomy.* Good value. Mixed quality questions with concise answers.

B **Anatomy** $17.95 Review/70 q

Oklahoma Notes, Papka

Springer-Verlag, 1995, 231 pages, ISBN 0387943951

Concise content review covers embryology, gross anatomy, neuroanatomy, and histology. Broad coverage, but format makes text difficult to read. Very few illustrations and tables. Limited student feedback.

B **Liebman's Neuroanatomy Made Easy & Understandable** $30.00 Review/Few q

Gertz

Aspen, 1995, 176 pages, ISBN 0834207303

Old edition easy to read. Contains excellent diagrams. A fast, straightforward, high-yield review. Expensive. New edition not yet reviewed.

B⁻ **Cell Biology: Review for New National Boards** $25.00 Review/524 q

Adelman

J&S, 1995, 203 pages, ISBN 0963287389

Question-based review format like other J&S books. Covers classic topics in cell biology. Contains some high quality micrographs. Recycles some questions and illustrations from J&S *Anatomy*. Limited-yield topic.

B⁻ **Neuroscience** $17.95 Test/509 q

Pretest, Siegel

McGraw-Hill, 1996, 209 pages, ISBN 0070520828

Old edition has detailed questions and answers. Includes photographs of CT/MRIs and drawings of brain sections. Useful after studying from other sources. For the motivated. New edition not yet reviewed.

C⁺ **Cell Biology & Histology** $21.00 Review/500 q

BRS, Gartner

Williams & Wilkins, 1993, 377 pages, ISBN 068303426X

Nice format with good reproductions, but too detailed. Nineteen chapters of histology with detailed answers. For the motivated student. Third edition expected in early 1996.

C⁺ **Essentials of Human Embryology** $39.95 Review only

Moore

Mosby, 1988, 194 pages, ISBN 0941158977

Good illustrations, pretty fast reading. However, too expensive to justify for a low-yield topic. Does not emphasize boards topics. No practice questions.

Anatomy

REVIEW RESOURCES

Histology QuizBank Vol. 1 & 2   **$69.00**   Software/800+ q
Downing
Keyboard Publishing, 1995, ISBN 1573493171 (Mac), ISBN 1573493198
(Windows)
Database of boards-style questions arranged by subject area. Explanations
on demand. Questions cross-referenced to Junqueira Text Stack (sold sep-
arately). Expensive for limited-yield topic.

 Molecular Biology QuizBank   **$59.00**   Software/500+ q
Case Western Reserve
Keyboard Publishing, 1995, ISBN 1573493422 (Mac), ISBN 1573493430
(Windows)
Software database of board-style questions. Expensive for limited-yield
topic.

 Wheater's Functional Histology   **$54.95**   Review only
Burkitt
Churchill-Livingstone, 1993, 407 pages, ISBN 0443046913
Color atlas with pictures of normal histology and accompanying text. Not
directed to boards type review. May be more useful for photomicrograph-
based questions.

C   **Anatomy**   **$17.95**   Test/500 q
PreTest, April
McGraw-Hill, 1996, 220 pages, ISBN 0070520909
Old edition has difficult questions with detailed answers. Some illustra-
tions. Requires time commitment. New edition not yet reviewed.

C   **Basic Histology: Examination and Board Review**   **$24.95**   Review/1200+ q
Paulsen
Appleton & Lange, 1993, 407 pages, ISBN 0838505694
Dense, thorough review, but low yield for boards. Good format with many
questions. Designed to complement Junqueira's *Basic Histology* textbook.
Requires time commitment. New edition expected in 1996.

C   **Basic Histopathology**   **$54.95**   Review only
Wheater
Churchill-Livingstone, 1991, 252 pages, ISBN 0443042373
Color atlas with text. Contains pictures of pathological histology. Not di-
rected to boards-type review. May be more useful for photomicrograph-
based questions.

REVIEW RESOURCES

Anatomy

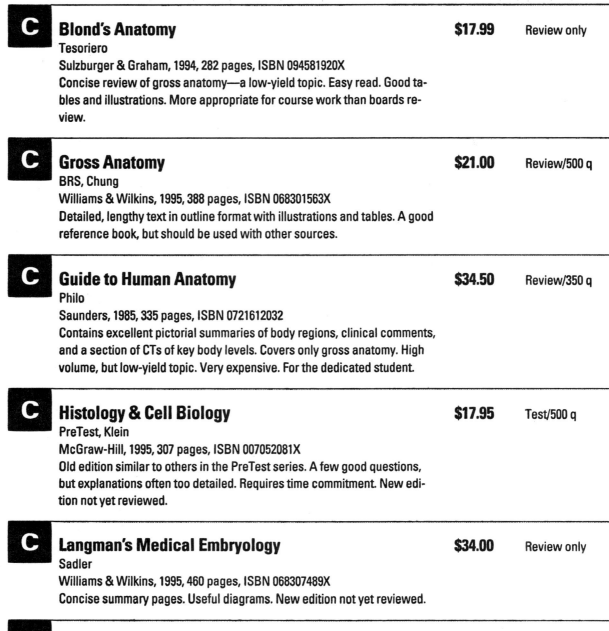

C **Blond's Anatomy**   **$17.99**   Review only
Tesoriero
Sulzburger & Graham, 1994, 282 pages, ISBN 094581920X
Concise review of gross anatomy—a low-yield topic. Easy read. Good tables and illustrations. More appropriate for course work than boards review.

C **Gross Anatomy**   **$21.00**   Review/500 q
BRS, Chung
Williams & Wilkins, 1995, 388 pages, ISBN 068301563X
Detailed, lengthy text in outline format with illustrations and tables. A good reference book, but should be used with other sources.

C **Guide to Human Anatomy**   **$34.50**   Review/350 q
Philo
Saunders, 1985, 335 pages, ISBN 0721612032
Contains excellent pictorial summaries of body regions, clinical comments, and a section of CTs of key body levels. Covers only gross anatomy. High volume, but low-yield topic. Very expensive. For the dedicated student.

C **Histology & Cell Biology**   **$17.95**   Test/500 q
PreTest, Klein
McGraw-Hill, 1995, 307 pages, ISBN 007052081X
Old edition similar to others in the PreTest series. A few good questions, but explanations often too detailed. Requires time commitment. New edition not yet reviewed.

C **Langman's Medical Embryology**   **$34.00**   Review only
Sadler
Williams & Wilkins, 1995, 460 pages, ISBN 068307489X
Concise summary pages. Useful diagrams. New edition not yet reviewed.

C **MedCharts: Anatomy**   **$17.95**   Review only
Gest
ILOC, 1994, 309 pages, ISBN 1882531019
Tabular summaries of gross anatomy for course and board review. Chart overkill is low yield.

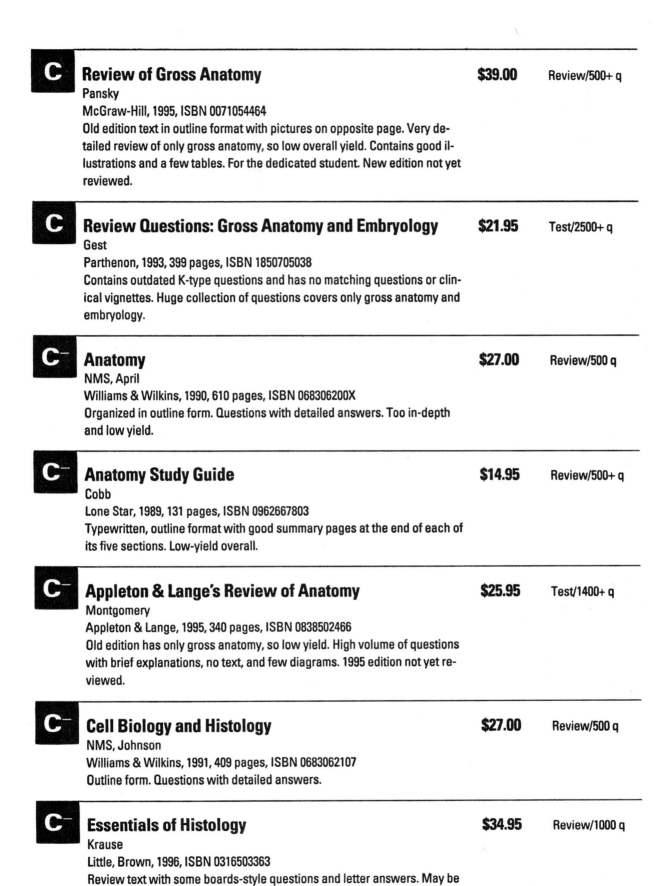

C **Review of Gross Anatomy**   **$39.00**   Review/500+ q

Pansky

McGraw-Hill, 1995, ISBN 0071054464

Old edition text in outline format with pictures on opposite page. Very detailed review of only gross anatomy, so low overall yield. Contains good illustrations and a few tables. For the dedicated student. New edition not yet reviewed.

C **Review Questions: Gross Anatomy and Embryology**   **$21.95**   Test/2500+ q

Gest

Parthenon, 1993, 399 pages, ISBN 1850705038

Contains outdated K-type questions and has no matching questions or clinical vignettes. Huge collection of questions covers only gross anatomy and embryology.

C⁻ **Anatomy**   **$27.00**   Review/500 q

NMS, April

Williams & Wilkins, 1990, 610 pages, ISBN 068306200X

Organized in outline form. Questions with detailed answers. Too in-depth and low yield.

C⁻ **Anatomy Study Guide**   **$14.95**   Review/500+ q

Cobb

Lone Star, 1989, 131 pages, ISBN 0962667803

Typewritten, outline format with good summary pages at the end of each of its five sections. Low-yield overall.

C⁻ **Appleton & Lange's Review of Anatomy**   **$25.95**   Test/1400+ q

Montgomery

Appleton & Lange, 1995, 340 pages, ISBN 0838502466

Old edition has only gross anatomy, so low yield. High volume of questions with brief explanations, no text, and few diagrams. 1995 edition not yet reviewed.

C⁻ **Cell Biology and Histology**   **$27.00**   Review/500 q

NMS, Johnson

Williams & Wilkins, 1991, 409 pages, ISBN 0683062107

Outline form. Questions with detailed answers.

C⁻ **Essentials of Histology**   **$34.95**   Review/1000 q

Krause

Little, Brown, 1996, ISBN 0316503363

Review text with some boards-style questions and letter answers. May be more appropriate as a course text than review book. New edition not yet reviewed.

Gross Anatomy: A Review with Questions and Explanations

$28.95   Review/430+ q

Snell
Little, Brown, 1990, 345 pages, ISBN 0316801976
A preeminent author. Dense, thorough, and requires time commitment.
Good diagrams. Some questions outdated. Very little clinical correlation.
Still low yield.

MEPC Histology

$40.00   Review/300 q

Amenta
Appleton & Lange, 1995, 94 pages, ISBN 1572350695
Old edition very detailed for low-yield topic. Very expensive. New edition
not yet reviewed.

Human Developmental Anatomy

$27.00   Review/450 q

NMS, Johnson
Williams & Wilkins, 1989, 447 pages, ISBN 0683062263
Outline form. Low yield.

Keyboard Histology Series Personal Edition

$149.00   Software/800+ q

Keyboard Publishing, 1995, ISBN 1573492973 (Mac), ISBN 1573492981
(Windows)
Includes Histology Quizbanks Vol. 1 & 2 (reviewed above) and Junqueira
Histology Text Stack. Quizbank questions linked to passages in Text Stack.
Text can be exported to word processor. Very expensive for a limited-yield
subject. Better if purchased by the library. Text Stack more appropriate for
reference than review.

Neuroanatomy

$27.00   Review/300 q

NMS, DeMyer
Williams & Wilkins, 1990, 380 pages, ISBN 0683062360
Outline form. Too detailed. Nice diagrams, but low yield.

Neuroanatomy

$21.95   Review/500 q

BRS, Fix
Williams & Wilkins, 1995, 416 pages, ISBN 0683032496
Updated text. Covers anatomy and embryology of the nervous system. Still
low yield.

Anatomy

REVIEW RESOURCES

Neuroanatomy: A Review with Questions and Explanations
Snell
Little, Brown, 1992, 298 pages, ISBN 0316802468
Reasonably easy to read, contains some clinical correlations. Length of the book too long relative to the small portion of the exam related to neuroanatomy.

$29.95   Review/400+ q

Student Aid to Gross Anatomy
Snell
Appleton & Lange, 1986, 514 pages, ISBN 0838586872
A pocket-sized handbook for quick reference. Written as an abstract of the larger textbook, which covers gross anatomy by system. Good organization but too detailed for the boards.

$19.50   Review only

NEW BOOKS—ANATOMY

Mosby Ace Anatomy
Moore
Mosby-Year Book, 1996, ISBN 0815169051
Expected in early 1996. Concise content review with boards-style questions. Test software included with text. Money-back guarantee.

$25.95   Review/600+ q

Mosby Ace Histology & Cell Biology
Burns
Mosby-Year Book, 1996, ISBN 0815113382
Expected in early 1996. Concise content review with boards-style questions. Test software included with text. Money-back guarantee.

$25.95   Review/600+ q

Mosby Ace Neuroanatomy
Castro
Mosby-Year Book, 1996, ISBN 0815114796
Expected in early 1996. Concise content review with boards-style questions. Test software included with text. Money-back guarantee.

$28.95   Review/600+ q

PreTest Anatomy Study Disk
April
McGraw-Hill, 1995, ISBN 0078641632 (Mac), ISBN 0078641624 (Windows)
Software test review based on *PreTest Anatomy* text. Includes questions with detailed answers and some illustrations. Program can custom-generate tests. Copy protection mechanism is inconvenient.

$28.00   Software/500 q

REVIEW RESOURCES

Anatomy

A **Behavioral Science Review** $21.95 Review/500 q

BRS, Fadem

Williams & Wilkins, 1994, 237 pages, ISBN 0683029533

Easy reading, outline format, boldfacing of key terms. Appropriate length
and good detailed coverage of high-yield topics. Great tables and charts.
Quick review. Good value.

B⁺ **Behavioral Science** $27.00 Review/325 q

NMS, Wiener

Williams & Wilkins, 1995, 375 pages, ISBN 0683062034

New edition retains detailed multidisciplinary outline, but with improved
formatting. Neatly organized. Incorporates DSM-IV. Probably more detailed
than necessary. For the motivated student starting early or to be used as a
reference. New biostatistics chapter is inadequate.

B **Behavioral Sciences for the Boreds** $14.95 Review only

Sierles

MedMaster, 1993, 146 pages, ISBN 0940780194

Short, easy reading, reasonable yield, but can get lost in narrative format.
Includes biostatistics, medical sociology, psychopathology. Not enough to
achieve a high score. Must supplement with another text. Casual style
does not appeal to all students. Appropriate if you have very limited time.

B **High-Yield Biostatistics** $15.00 Review only

Glaser

Williams & Wilkins, 1995, 83 pages, ISBN 0683035665

Complete, well-written, illustrated book covering the biostatistics likely to
be on the USMLE Step 1. Good review exercises. Still, limited-yield topic.
For the motivated student, not for last-minute cramming.

B **Review of Epidemiology and Biostatistics** $21.95 Review

Hanrahan

Appleton & Lange, 1994, 109 pages, ISBN 083850244X

Excellent, concise overview of epidemiology with complete explanations
and diagrams. Does not include other behavioral science subtopics. Expensive and limited yield. Good for the motivated student.

B⁻ **Behavioral Sciences** $17.95 Review/145+ q

Oklahoma Notes, Krug

Springer-Verlag, 1995, 311 pages, ISBN 0387943935

Typewritten, easy reading. Outline format. Questions of mixed quality. Good
tables. For the motivated student.

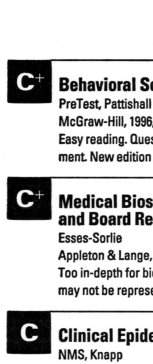

C+ Behavioral Sciences

$17.95   Test/500 q

PreTest, Pattishall
McGraw-Hill, 1996, 275 pages, ISBN 0070520844
Easy reading. Questions with detailed answers. Requires some time invest-
ment. New edition not yet reviewed.

C+ Medical Biostatistics and Epidemiology: Examination and Board Review

$26.95   Review

Esses-Sorlie
Appleton & Lange, 1995, 359 pages, ISBN 0838562191
Too in-depth for biostatistics. Requires time commitment. Sample questions
may not be representative of the USMLE Step 1.

C Clinical Epidemiology and Biostatistics

$27.00   Review/300 q

NMS, Knapp
Williams & Wilkins, 1992, 435 pages, ISBN 0683062069
Overkill for a limited-yield topic.

C− Psychiatry Made Ridiculously Simple

$11.95   Review only

Good
MedMaster, 1995, 90 pages, ISBN 0940780224
Easy reading. Includes epidemiology. Low basic science yield, but very
good clinical material.

NEW BOOKS—BEHAVIORAL SCIENCE

A Review of Biostatistics

$22.95   Review only

Leaverton
Little, Brown, 1995, 117 pages, ISBN 0316518832
Complete review of biostatistics. Not yet reviewed.

Digging Up the Bones: Behavioral Sciences

$16.00   Review only

Linardakis
Michaelis Medical, 1995, 85 pages, ISBN 1884084001
New high-yield review of behavioral science. Limited student feedback.

Mosby Ace Behavioral Science

$24.95   Review/600+ q

Cody
Mosby-Year Book, 1996, ISBN 0815118449
Expected in early 1996. Concise content review with boards-style ques-
tions. Test software included with text. Money-back guarantee.

Behavioral Science

REVIEW RESOURCES

A Lippincott's Illustrated Reviews: Biochemistry $29.95 Review/250+ q
Champe
Lippincott, 1994, 443 pages, ISBN 0397510918
Excellent diagrams. Emphasizes concepts. Good clinical correlations. Comprehensive review of biochemistry, including low-yield topics. Excellent book, but requires time commitment, so must start early. Best used while taking the course.

A⁻ Biochemistry $21.95 Review/500 q
BRS, Marks
Williams & Wilkins, 1994, 337 pages, ISBN 0683055976
Easy-to-read outline with very good boldfaced chapter summaries. More concise alternative to Lippincott. Outline format not ideal for some sections. Mixed-quality diagrams. High-yield clinical correlations at end of each chapter. Questions with short answers.

B⁺ Biochemistry: A Review with Questions and Explanations $28.95 Review/220+ q
Friedman
Little, Brown, 1995, 220 pages, ISBN 0316294284
Good quality, concise text review. Metabolism section is well illustrated. Molecular biochemistry section fails to emphasize important concepts and has few illustrations. Too few pathways; too many structures. Boards-style questions favor basic biochemistry over clinical correlation. Letter answers with occasional short explanations.

B⁺ Biochemistry: Review for New National Boards $25.00 Test/505 q
Kumar
J & S, 1993, 211 pages, ISBN 0963287311
Quick review of biochemistry consisting primarily of questions with detailed answers. Includes clinical vignettes and extended matching questions; few diagrams. Use in conjunction with other resources.

B⁺ Digging Up the Bones: Biochemistry $16.00 Review only
Wilson
Michaelis Medical, 1994, 124 pages, ISBN 1884084044
Collection of high-yield biochemistry facts. Use for last-minute review or in conjunction with another review book.

B **Biochemistry**   **$17.95**   Review/530+ q
Oklahoma Notes, Briggs
Springer-Verlag, 1995, 287 pages, ISBN 0387943986
Dense text retains many hand-drawn diagrams. Good chapter on medical
genetics. Nonclinically oriented questions with brief explanations in the
margin. Multiple authors, inconsistent style. Limited student feedback.

B **Biochemistry**   **$17.95**   Test/500 q
PreTest, Chlapowski
McGraw-Hill, 1996, 231 pages, ISBN 0070520895
Old edition has difficult questions but good, detailed explanations. Referenced to biochemistry textbooks by Rawn and Stryer. Better than average
for this series. Use to strengthen knowledge after reviewing biochemistry
through other means. New edition not yet reviewed.

B **Biochemistry: Examination and Board Review**   **$28.95**   Review/500+ q
Balcavage
Appleton & Lange, 1995, 433 pages, ISBN 0838506615
Comprehensive review of biochemistry. Requires time commitment. Appro-
priate as a course text. Has some clinical correlations.

B **Biochemistry Illustrated**   **$34.95**   Review only
Campbell
Churchill-Livingstone, 1994, 304 pages, ISBN 0443045739
Excellent diagrams with explanations but no questions. Good for students
who prefer learning by diagrams. Readable. Very expensive. Requires time
commitment.

B **Blond's Biochemistry**   **$17.99**   Review only
Guttenplan
Sulzburger & Graham, 1994, 269 pages, ISBN 0945819498
Easy reading. Moderate time commitment. Some topics covered only su-
perficially. Not boards oriented; may be more appropriate with coursework.

B **Clinical Biochemistry Made Ridiculously Simple**   **$21.95**   Review only
Goldberg
MedMaster, 1993, 93 pages, ISBN 0940780100
Conceptual approach to clinical biochemistry, with humor. The casual style
does not appeal to all students. A good overview and integration for all
metabolic pathways. Includes a 23-page clinical review that is very high-
yield and crammable. Contains a unique fold-out "road map" of
metabolism. Not adequate as sole study source. For students with firm biochemistry background.

B Metabolism at a Glance

$24.95   Review only

Salway

Blackwell Science, 1994, 95 pages, ISBN 0632032588

Highly visual. Features diagrams with associated text. Illustrations pretty but complicated. Use as a supplement to traditional review books. Large-page format.

B⁻ Biochemistry

$27.00   Review/500 q

NMS, Davidson

Williams & Wilkins, 1994, 584 pages, ISBN 0683062050

Very long, detailed outline. Questions with detailed answers. Good pathway illustrations but too much chemical structure detail. Concise review of genetics. Overall, too detailed to use as review text unless previously used during coursework. For the motivated student.

B⁻ MEPC Biochemistry

$16.95   Test/700 q

Glick

Appleton & Lange, 1995, 228 pages ISBN 0838557791

Picky questions with brief explanations. Revised edition has few clinical vignettes.

C⁺ Essentials of Biochemistry

$32.95   Review/100 q

Schumm

Little, Brown, 1995, 382 pages, ISBN 0316775312

Review text with some boards-style questions and letter answers. May be more appropriate as a course text than review book.

C⁺ Genetics

$27.00   Review/300 q

NMS, Friedman

Williams & Wilkins, 1995, ISBN 0683062174

Old edition has detailed outline format supplemented by numerous charts and diagrams. Low yield. Some chapters not relevant for board review. For the very motivated student. New edition not yet reviewed.

C Basic Concepts in Biochemistry: A Student's Survival Guide

$25.95   Review only

Gilbert

McGraw-Hill, 1992, 298 pages, ISBN 0070234493

Presents concise summaries of difficult biochemical concepts and principles. Since it ignores much of the high-yield material, it is not very useful for boards review. Oriented toward undergraduate courses.

Genetics $17.95 Test/500 q
PreTest, Finkelstein
McGraw-Hill, 1996, 206 pages, ISBN 0070520836
Old edition has detailed questions and answers. Questions of mixed quality
Limited student feedback. New edition not yet reviewed.

NEW BOOKS—BIOCHEMISTRY

Mosby Ace Biochemistry $27.95 Review/600+ q
Wurzel
Mosby-Year Book, 1996, ISBN 0815192762
Expected in late 1996. Concise content review with boards-style questions.
Test software included with text. Money-back guarantee.

PreTest Biochemistry Study Disk $28.00 Software/500 q
Chlapowski
McGraw-Hill, 1995, ISBN 0078641659 (Mac), ISBN 0078641640 (Windows)
Software test review based on *PreTest Biochemistry*. Includes questions
with detailed answers and some illustrations. Program can custom-
generate tests. Copy protection mechanism is inconvenient.

Biochemistry

REVIEW RESOURCES

Medical Microbiology & Immunology: Examination and Board Review

$28.95   Review/692 q

Levinson

Appleton & Lange, 1994, 491 pages, ISBN 0838562426

Clear, concise writing, with excellent diagrams and tables. Excellent yield for both text and questions. Forty-two page "Summary of Medically Important Organisms" very crammable. Requires time commitment. Good practice questions but with letter answers only. Highest overall student rating for any board review book. New edition expected in early 1996.

Microbiology: Review for New National Boards

$25.00   Test/507 q

Stokes

J & S, 1993, 194 pages, ISBN 096328732X

Easy reading. Covers many high-yield topics and includes case-based questions and extended matching questions. Very good question-and-answer-based review of clinically relevant microbiology, but lacking somewhat in detailed information. Excellent supplement to a review book.

Clinical Microbiology Made Ridiculously Simple

$21.95   Review

Gladwin

MedMaster, 1995, 268 pages, ISBN 0940780208

Good review of microbiology. Clever and humorous mnemonics. Text easy to read. Good tables and charts. Excellent antibiotic review. "Ridiculous" style does not appeal to everyone. Does not cover immunology.

Microbiology & Immunology

$21.95   Review/500 q

BRS, Johnson

Williams & Wilkins, 1993, 284 pages, ISBN 0683044656

Outline format, well organized. Good questions at the end of chapters. Too few diagrams. Updated for USMLE. Chapters on bacterial genetics and laboratory methods. Immunology section concise.

Appleton & Lange's Review of Microbiology and Immunology for USMLE Step 1

$26.95   Test/995 q

Yotis

Appleton & Lange, 1993, 216 pages, ISBN 0838500595

Questions with detailed answers. Updated for the USMLE. Well referenced. Inadequate as a primary source, but a very good supplement. For the motivated student.

REVIEW RESOURCES

Microbiology

B+ Microbiology

$27.95 Review only

Tof

Alert and Oriented, 1994, 243 pages, ISBN 0964012413

Chart format is well organized and easy to read and carry. Most relevant to micro topics. High-yield flash cards are a plus. Has a short immunology review.

B Buzzwords in Microbiology

$19.95 Review only

Hurst

Bryan Edwards, 1994, 155 pages, ISBN 1878576089

Spiral-bound flash cards contain important facts about the most medically relevant bacteria and fungi. Directed to boards review. Bullet presentation of information affords easy and quick review. Excellent pictures and buzzwords. Useful as a speedy pocket-sized review after studying from a more complete text. Does not cover virology, parasitology, and immunology.

B Medical Microbiology: A Review with Questions and Explanations

$29.95 Review/450+ q

Hentges

Little, Brown, 1995, 288 pages, ISBN 0316357847

Comprehensive review takes time commitment. Revised edition has updated tables and charts. Improved format and organization. Summation chapter at end of book is of limited value. Limited student feedback.

B Microbiology and Immunology

$17.95 Review/300+ q

Oklahoma Notes, Hyde

Springer-Verlag, 1995, 229 pages, ISBN 0387943927

Old edition easy to read, but not adequate as sole study source. Good summary statements at end of each chapter. Extended matching questions. Poor typeface and diagrams. Unequal coverage. New edition not yet reviewed.

B− Blond's Microbiology

$15.99 Review only

Alcamo

Sulzberger & Graham, 1994, 181 pages, ISBN 0945819412

Text review. Spotty coverage of some key topics. Below average for this series.

B− Digging Up the Bones: Microbiology

$16.00 Review only

Linardakis

Michaelis Medical, 1993, 99 pages, ISBN 188408401X

Old edition easy to read. Brief collection of phrases and associations based on answers to assorted multiple-choice questions. A few tables and simple diagrams. Very expensive for the amount of material. New edition not yet reviewed.

Essential Immunology Review

$19.95   Test/422 q

Roitt

Blackwell Scientific, 1995, 319 pages, ISBN 0865424586

Boards-style questions with explanations that also discuss the incorrect answers.

Immunology at a Glance

$24.95   Review only

Playfair

Blackwell Scientific, 1992, 43 pages, ISBN 0632033150

Diagram-based synopsis of immunology. Text and figures on the left, with legends on the right. Expensive for length of book.

MEPC Microbiology

$19.95   Test/700 q

Kim

Appleton & Lange, 1995, 257 pages, ISBN 0838563082

Updated with clinical vignettes. Good infectious disease questions. Variable quality questions. Easy read. Explanations are brief and direct.

Microbiology

$27.00   Review/500 q

NMS, Kingsbury

Williams & Wilkins, 1990, 436 pages, ISBN 0683062344

Outline form. Too detailed in some areas. Insufficient immunology; NMS has a separate immunology book. Lacks good explanation of bacterial genetics. Updated material on AIDS. Useful only if previously used as a textbook.

Microbiology

$17.95   Test/500 q

PreTest, Tilton

McGraw-Hill, 1996, 191 pages, ISBN 0070520003

Old edition has mixed-quality questions with detailed explanations. Questions often too difficult and answers verbose. New edition not yet reviewed.

Microbiology QuizBanks Vol. 2 & 3

$69.00   Software/800+ q

Gotts

Keyboard Publishing, 1995, ISBN 1573493252 (Mac), 1573493279 (Windows)

Computer-based questions with explanations. Questions electronically referenced to Sherris Microbiology Text Stack (sold separately). Available for PC and Mac. Expensive.

Immunology

$27.00   Review/300 q

NMS, Hyde

Williams & Wilkins, 1995, 316 pages, ISBN 068306231X

Outline form. Very detailed. Good figures and explanations of laboratory methods. Updated information on immune response, but lengthy for immunology alone. Requires time commitment.

Immunology QuizBank Vol. 1

$69.00   Software/400+ q

Roitt

Keyboard Publishing, 1995, ISBN 157349321X (Mac), 1573493236 (Windows)

Software database of boards-style questions with explanations. Questions electronically referenced to Roitt Immunology Text Stack (sold separately). Packaged with bonus case collection. Very expensive for number of questions.

The Keyboard Immunology Series Personal Edition

$149.00   Software/400 q

Roitt

Keyboard Publishing, 1995, ISBN 1573492035 (Mac), ISBN 1573492043 (Windows).

More appropriate for use with coursework. Includes Histology QuizBank and *Essential Immunology* Text Stack by Roitt. Questions cross-linked to Text Stack. Text can be exported to a word processor. Available for PC and Macintosh. Limited student feedback. Good learning tool but beyond the student budget. More appropriate as a library purchase.

The Keyboard Microbiology Series Personal Edition

$149.00   Software/800 q

Ryan

Keyboard Publishing, 1995, ISBN 1573492701 (Mac), ISBN 157349271X (Windows)

Includes two Microbiology QuizBanks and the electronic edition of *Sherris Medical Microbiology*. Questions cross-linked to Text Stack. Text can be exported to a word processor. More appropriate for use with course work and as a reference. Good learning tool but beyond the student budget. More appropriate as a library purchase.

Microbiology & Immunology Casebook

$18.95   Review/185 q

Barrett

Little, Brown, 1995, 262 pages, ISBN 0316081329

Uses case examples to cover major concepts. Cases do not resemble typical boards vignettes. Useful only as a supplement to a review book.

Immunology Illustrated Outline

$19.95   Review only

Male

Raven Press, 1991, ISBN 0397448252

Pocket-sized booklet, well organized, concise. Quick to read and review

Not targeted for boards review.

NEW BOOKS—MICROBIOLOGY

Lippincott's Illustrated Reviews: Microbiology

—   Review

Strohl

Lippincott, 1996

Expected in 1996. Features a comprehensive, highly illustrated review of microbiology similar in style to Champe's *Lippincott Biochemistry*.

Micro Charts

$24.95   Review only

Weiner

MRO MicroCharts, 1993, 116 pages

Not yet reviewed. Quick review of microbiology in tabular form.

Mosby Ace Microbiology & Immunology

$28.95   Review/600+ q

Rosenthal

Mosby-Year Book, 1996, ISBN 0815173490

Expected in early 1996. Features a concise content review with boards-style questions. Test software included with text. Money-back guarantee.

PreTest Microbiology Study Disk

$28.00   Software/500 q

Tilton

McGraw-Hill, 1995, ISBN 0078641551 (Mac), ISBN 0078641543 (Windows)

Software test review based on *PreTest Microbiology* text. Includes questions with detailed answers and some illustrations. Program can custom-generate tests. Copy protection mechanism is inconvenient.

REVIEW RESOURCES

Microbiology

Pathology

$21.95   Review/500 q

BRS, Schneider

Williams & Wilkins, 1993, 412 pages, ISBN 0683076086

Excellent, concise review with appropriate emphasis. Outline format chapters with boldfacing of key facts. Excellent questions with explanations at the end of each chapter. Well-organized tables and diagrams. Good black-and-white photographs representative of classic pathology. Consistently high student recommendations.

Introduction to Clinical Pathophysiology

$29.95   Review/few q.

McPhee

Appleton & Lange, 1995, 512 pages, ISBN 0838578152

New interdisciplinary course text that students report is useful in dealing with the growing clinical slant of the boards. Excellent integration of basic sciences with mechanisms of disease. Does not discuss pharmacotherapy. Few non-boards-style questions.

Pathology: Review for New National Boards

$25.00   Test/509 q

Miller

J & S, 1993, 222 pages, ISBN 0963287338

Question-and-answer-based review of pathology. Includes many case-based questions. Focuses on high-yield topics. Good black-and-white photographs. Inadequate as sole source of review. Expensive for number of questions.

Appleton & Lange's Review of General Pathology

$26.95   Test/896 q

Lewis

Appleton & Lange, 1993, 197 pages, ISBN 0838501613

Short text sections followed by lots of questions with answers. Some very useful high-yield tables at the beginning of each section. Good illustrations and photographs. Covers only general pathology (i.e., no organ-based pathology). Can be used as a supplement to more detailed texts. Reviewable in a short period.

Medical Exam Review: Pathology

$21.95   Test/600 q

A&L/MEPC, Fayemi

Appleton & Lange, 1994, 317 pages, ISBN 0838584411

Good-quality questions with explanations. Good case-study chapter. Use as a supplement to other review books.

REVIEW RESOURCES

Pathology

B⁺ **Pathology Notes** $24.95 Review only

Chandrasoma

Appleton & Lange, 1992, 788 pages, ISBN 0838551645

Lengthy, but well organized and easy to read. Requires considerable time commitment. Good tables, no photographs. Good line drawings. Compare the format with Pocket Companion to Robbins as to which best suits your style. Companion to *Concise Pathology* by same authors.

B⁺ **Pocket Companion to Robbins' Pathologic Basis of Diseases** $25.00 Review only

Robbins

Saunders, 1995, 620 pages, ISBN 0721657427

Old edition was good for reviewing associations between keywords and specific diseases. Very condensed, easy to understand. Explains most important diseases and pathologic processes. No photographs or illustrations. Useful as a quick reference. New edition not yet reviewed.

B **Digging Up the Bones: Pathology** $16.00 Review only

Linardakis

Michaelis Medical, 1993, 106 pages, ISBN 1884084028

Easy reading. Brief collection of phrases and associations often based on answers to assorted multiple-choice questions. Very expensive for the amount of material. New edition expected in early 1996.

B **Pathology** $17.95 Review/140 q

Oklahoma Notes, Holliman

Springer-Verlag, 1995, 279 pages, ISBN 0387943900

Dense text. Few diagrams and tables. No illustrations. Questions with letter answers only. Good when you have no time for comprehensive review books. New edition not yet reviewed.

B **Pathology: Examination and Board Review** $26.95 Review

Newland

Appleton & Lange, 1995, 314 pages, ISBN 0838577199

Moderate text review with many high-quality illustrations. Has some good charts and illustrations. Some overlap with microbiology. Limited student feedback.

B **Pathology Illustrated** $54.95 Review only

Govan

Churchill-Livingstone, 1995, 843 pages, ISBN 0443050686

Lengthy, but fast reading. Well-illustrated with many line drawings. User-friendly format. Worth considering despite price. New edition not reviewed.

Pathology

REVIEW RESOURCES

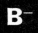

Neuropathology and Basic Neuroscience

$17.95   Review/101 q

Oklahoma Notes, Brumback
Springer-Verlag, 1995, 289 pages, ISBN 0387943897
Utilizes organ system approach by integrating CNS anatomy, pathology, physiology, and some pharmacology. Easy to read. Good quality line drawings. Use either with organ system review or as a supplement to a subject review. Limited student feedback.

Pathologic Basis of Disease Self-Assessment and Review

$21.75   Test/1600+ q

Compton
Saunders, 1995, 239 pages, ISBN 0721640419
Old edition features huge number of good practice questions, some very difficult and detailed. A good buy for the number of questions. Includes outdated K-type question format. Very good for the dedicated student. New edition not yet reviewed.

Pathology

$27.00   Review/500 q

NMS, LiVolsi
Williams & Wilkins, 1994, 508 pages, ISBN 0683062433
Outline form. Comprehensive review of large amount of material. Sometimes too detailed. Slow reading.

Pathology Facts

$19.95   Review only

Harruff
Lippincott, 1994, 424 pages, ISBN 0397512589
A handbook-size text database, organized by disease. Limited topic coverage. Worth considering.

Pathology QuizBank, Vol. 2

$99.00   Software/1,000+ q

Faculty UC Davis
Keyboard Publishing, 1995, ISBN 1573493295 (Mac), ISBN 1573493317 (Windows)
Expensive software database of board-style questions with explanations. Electronically referenced to Robbins Pathology Text Stack. Quizzer has no timer or ability to custom-generate tests.

Pathology

$17.95   Test/500 q

PreTest, Brown
McGraw-Hill, 1996, 299 pages, ISBN 0070520860
Old edition has difficult questions with detailed, complete answers. Often obscure or esoteric questions. Good-quality photographs. Can be used as a supplement to other review books. For the motivated student. New edition revised by new editor; not yet reviewed.

The Keyboard Pathology Series Personal Edition

$199.00 Software/1000+ q

Cotran

Keyboard Publishing, 1995, ISBN 1573492116 (Mac), ISBN 1573492124 (Windows)

Includes electronic edition of the 5th edition of Robbins' *Pathologic Basis of Disease* on CD-ROM and *Pathology QuizBank*. Very good if used as reference or with course. Beyond the student budget. More appropriate as a library purchase.

Review of Pathophysiology

$40.00 Review/130 q

Kaufman

Little, Brown, 1983, 555 pages, ISBN 0316483397

Relatively easy to read, with outline format and diagrams. Appropriate for the student establishing a solid base in clinical pathophysiology, but not directly relevant to the boards. New edition expected in 1996.

NEW BOOKS—PATHOLOGY

Essentials of Pathophysiology

$34.95 Review/100 q

Kaufman

Little, Brown, 1996, ISBN 0316484059

Expected in early 1996. Review text with some boards-style questions and letter answers. Compare to the McPhee *Introduction to Clinical Pathophysiology* book.

Mosby Ace Pathology

$27.95 Text/600+ q

Pelley

Mosby-Year Book, 1996, ISBN 0815173490

Expected in late 1996. Features a concise content review with boards-style questions. Test software included with text. Money-back guarantee.

PreTest Pathology Study Disk

$28.00 Software/500 q

Brown

McGraw-Hill, 1995, ISBN 0078641594 (Mac); ISBN 0078641586 (Windows)

Software test review based on *PreTest Pathology.* Includes questions with detailed answers and some illustrations. Program can custom-generate tests. Copy protection mechanism is convenient.

A

Pharmacology: Examination and Board Review

$24.95   Review/650+ q

Katzung

Appleton & Lange, 1995, 509 pages, ISBN 083858067X

High-yield text is well organized and easy to read. Good charts and tables.
Relevant questions with concise explanations. Good for drug interactions
and toxicities. Good diagrams and a crammable list of "top boards drugs."

A⁻

Lippincott's Illustrated Reviews: Pharmacology

$29.95   Review/230+ q

Harvey

Lippincott, 1992, 459 pages, ISBN 039751039X

Outline format with practice questions and many excellent illustrations and
tables. Cross-referenced to Lippincott's *Biochemistry*. Includes outdated K-
type questions. Detailed, so must start early. For the motivated student.
New edition expected June 1996.

B⁺

Clinical Pharmacology Made Ridiculously Simple

$17.95   Review only

Olson

MedMaster, 1994, 162 pages, ISBN 0940780178

Includes general principles and many drug summary charts. Particularly
strong in cardiovascular drugs and antimicrobials, incomplete in other areas. The casual style does not work for some students. Well-organized, but
sometimes too detailed. Effective as a chart-based review book but not as
a sole study source. Must supplement with a more detailed text.

B

Blond's Pharmacology

$19.99   Review only

Kostrzewa

Sulzburger & Graham, 1995, 398 pages, ISBN 094581948X

Concise review of pharmacology. Many good diagrams. Some key topics
inadequately covered.

B

MEPC Pharmacology

$16.95   Test/700 q

Krzanowski

Appleton & Lange, 1995, 267 pages, ISBN 0838562272

Questions with brief, direct explanation. Well referenced. Answers recently
updated.

B

Medical Pharmacology at a Glance

$24.95   Review only

Neal

Blackwell Science, 1992, 92 pages, ISBN 0632033738

Contains excellent figures followed by explanations. Visual synthesis of
sites and mechanisms of drug actions. Occasionally, British terminology
may be confusing. High yield for those with limited study time. Useful only
as a supplement to a review text. May be hard to find.

REVIEW RESOURCES

Pharmacology

B Pharmacology

$17.95   Test/500 q

PreTest, DiPalma

McGraw-Hill, 1996, 253 pages, ISBN 0070520879

Old edition is typical for this series. Questions are somewhat difficult with detailed answers. For the motivated student. Above average for series. New edition not yet reviewed.

B Pharmacology

$27.00   Review/300+ q

NMS, Jacob

Williams & Wilkins, 1996, 373 pages, ISBN 0683062514

Old edition features outline format. Not enough tables. Often too detailed. Lacks emphasis on high-yield material. Has a lengthy USMLE-type exam. Reflects updated treatments of AIDS, Lyme disease, and other topics. Requires time commitment. New edition not yet reviewed.

B Pharmacology

$17.95   Review/560+ q

Oklahoma Notes, Moore

Springer-Verlag, 1995, 235 pages, ISBN 0387943943

Conceptual approach. Features USMLE-type questions with brief explanations. A concise and readable review book.

B Pharmacology: A Review with Questions and Answers

$27.95   Review/400+ q

Ebadi

Little, Brown, 1996, ISBN 0316199575

Old edition very long, requires time commitment. Tables are somewhat difficult to use. Includes clinical case-based questions. New edition not yet reviewed.

B⁻ Digging Up the Bones: Pharmacology

$16.00   Review only

Linardakis

Michaelis Medical, 1993, 85 pages, ISBN 1884084001

Easy reading. Brief collection of phrases and associations based on answers to assorted multiple-choice questions. Very expensive for the amount of material. Below average for series. New edition expected in early 1996.

B⁻ Med Charts, Pharmacology

$14.95   Review only

Rosenbach

ILOC, 1993, 171 pages, ISBN 1882531000

Contains tables and summaries. Good for quick review, but requires previous reading from other sources. May be helpful for students who prefer studying charts.

Pharmacology
B⁻

BRS, Rosenfeld
Williams & Wilkins, 1993, 357 pages, ISBN 0683073613
Outline format. Good use of boldface, although few tables. Questions are of moderate difficulty with short answers.

$21.00 Review/450 q

The Pharmacology Text Stack Personal Edition
C⁺

Theoharides
Keyboard Publishing 1993, ISBN 1573492132 (Mac), ISBN 1573492140 (Windows)
Includes text of electronic pharmacology textbook by Theoharides. Questions linked to text. Good as reference or with course. Too expensive for students. More appropriate as a library purchase.

$135.00 Software/200+ q

NEW BOOKS—PHARMACOLOGY

Essentials of Pharmacology

Theoharides
Little, Brown, 1996, ISBN 0316839361
Review text with some boards-style questions and letter answers. May be more appropriate as a course text than review book. New edition expected in early 1996.

$29.95 Review/100 q

Mosby Ace Pharmacology

Enna
Mosby-Year Book 1996, ISBN 0815131127
Expected in early 1996. Concise content review with boards-style questions. Test software included with text. Money-back guarantee.

$28.95 Review/600+ q

Pharmacology: Review for New National Boards

Billingsley
J & S, 1995, 186 pages, ISBN 0963287370
Not yet reviewed. Questions with explanations. Follows format of other J & S books.

$25.00 Test/539 q

PreTest Pharmacology Study Disk

DiPalma
McGraw-Hill, 1995, ISBN 0078641616 (Mac), ISBN 0078641608 (Windows)
Software test review based on *PreTest Pharmacology*. Includes questions with detailed answers and some illustrations. Program can custom-generate tests. Copy protection mechanism is inconvenient.

$28.00 Software/500 q

Pharmacology

REVIEW RESOURCES

A

Physiology   **$21.95**   Review/400 q

BRS, Costanzo

Williams & Wilkins, 1995, 280 pages, ISBN 0683021346

Clear, concise review of physiology. Fast, easy reading. Great charts and tables. Good practice questions with explanations. Excellent review book, but may not be enough for in-depth coursework.

B⁺

Clinical Physiology Made Ridiculously Simple   **$17.95**   Review only

Goldberg

MedMaster, 1995, 152 pages, ISBN 0940780216

Easy reading with many "ridiculous" associations. Style does not work for everyone. Not as well illustrated as the rest of series.

B⁺

Physiology: An Illustrated Review with Questions & Explanations   **$27.95**   Review/320 q

Tadlock

Little, Brown, 1995, 333 pages, ISBN 0316827649

New edition features updated text with good illustrations and tables. Format and organization improved. Requires time commitment. Limited student feedback on new edition.

B

Blond's Physiology   **$20.00**   Review only

Grossman

Sulburger & Graham, 1995, 439 pages, ISBN 0945819420

Comprehensive but easy-to-read review text of physiology. Excellent diagrams and charts. Better than average for this series. Limited student feedback.

B

Color Atlas of Physiology   **$29.00**   Review only

Despopoulos

Georg Thieme Verlag, 1991, 369 pages, ISBN 0865773823

Compact, with over 156 colorful but complicated diagrams on the right and dense explanatory text on the left. Some translation problems. A unique, highly visual approach worthy of consideration. Useful as an adjunct to other review books.

REVIEW RESOURCES

Physiology

B **Essentials of Human Physiology** $38.95   Review only

Ackerman

Mosby-Year Book, 1992, 387 pages, ISBN 1556641095

Excellent diagrams with succinct accompanying text. Good sections on integrative and cardiovascular physiology. Few boards-type questions. Not to be used as sole source of review. New edition expected in early 1996. Will be renamed *Mosby Ace Physiology* and will feature testing software and more practice questions.

B **Physiology** $27.00   Review/300 q

NMS, Bullock

Williams & Wilkins, 1995, 641 pages, ISBN 068306259X

Old edition features very complete text in outline form. Often too detailed, but some good diagrams. Moderately difficult questions with detailed answers. Provides some pathophysiology. More useful if used as a course text; too long as a review text. For the motivated student. New edition not yet reviewed.

B **Physiology** $17.95   Test/500 q

PreTest, Mulligan

McGraw-Hill, 1996, 228 pages, ISBN 0070520852

Old edition has good questions with detailed explanations. Some questions too difficult. May be useful for the motivated student following extensive review from other sources. New edition not yet reviewed.

B **Physiology: A Review for the New National Boards** $25.00   Test/506 q

Jakoi

J & S, 1994, 214 pages, ISBN 0963287346

Good review book, but inadequate as sole source of review. Below average for this series. Limited student feedback.

B⁻ **MEPC Physiology** $16.95   Test/700 q

Penney

Appleton & Lange, 1995, 257 pages, ISBN 0838562221

Questions with brief, direct answers. Recently revised. Good as an adjunct to other review texts.

B⁻ **Physiology** $17.95   Review/300+ q

Oklahoma Notes, Thies

Springer-Verlag, 1995, 280 pages, ISBN 0387943978

Dense text. Inconsistent quality of sections. Emphasizes general concepts. Boards-type questions with short answers. Some errors.

Appleton & Lange's Review of Physiology

— Test/1000 q

Penney

Appleton & Lange, 1996

Boards-style questions with letter answers and explanations. Expected
September 1996.

Essentials of Physiology

$34.95 Review/100 q

Sperelakis

Little, Brown, 1996, ISBN 0316806285

Old edition features review text with some boards-style questions and letter answers. May be more appropriate as a course text than review book.
New edition expected in early 1996.

PreTest Physiology Study Disk

$28.00 Software/500 q

Ryan

McGraw-Hill, 1995, ISBN 0078641578 (Mac), ISBN 007864156X (Windows)

Software test review based on *PreTest Physiology*. Includes questions with
detailed answers and some illustrations. Program can custom generate
tests. Copy protection mechanism is inconvenient.

REVIEW RESOURCES

Physiology

Physiology

REVIEW RESOURCES

Commercial Review Courses

ArcVentures
National Medical School Review
Northwestern Learning Center
Postgraduate Medical Review
The Princeton Review
Stanley H. Kaplan
Youel's Prep

Commercial preparation courses can be helpful for some students, but these courses are expensive and require significant time commitment. They are usually effective in organizing study material for students who feel overwhelmed by the volume of material. Note that the multi-week courses may be quite intense and thus leave limited time for independent study. Note that some commercial courses are designed for first-time test takers while other courses focus on students who are repeating the examination. Some courses focus on foreign medical graduates who want to take all three Steps in a limited amount of time.

ArcVentures Medical Education Services

ArcVentures Medical Education Services (MES) offers a series of live-lecture preparation courses for all three Steps of the USMLE. The 1996 Step 1 courses include 7- and 15-week reviews in Chicago, Houston, Los Angeles, Miami, New Jersey, New York City, Puerto Rico and Washington, D.C. ArcVentures, Inc., is a subsidiary of Rush-Presbyterian-St. Luke's Medical Center in Chicago, Illinois.

The structured Step 1 courses review the seven basic sciences, with emphasis on material most likely to be found on the exam. ArcVentures' courses use a live-lecture format, with concise study notes and computer-scored practice exams. ArcVentures recruits US medical school faculty, including authors of basic science and medical board review books, to teach in the Step 1 program.

Students enrolled in the 7- and 15-Week Step 1 courses undergo an extensive review of the basic sciences and participate in small group activities where students review concepts covered in the lectures. With the help of ArcVentures' Diagnostic Exam, students can pinpoint areas for improvement and sharpen their test-taking skills. The 7- and 15-week courses are conducted out of ArcVentures' six regional offices and in Puerto Rico. The INTENSEPREP Step 1 course is designed for second-year medical students taking Step 1 for the first time. This course is offered annually at selected US medical schools.

Costs range from $900 for the INTENSEPREP course to $5500 for the 15-week review course. To receive an application and more information on tuition and course locations, call 1-800-860-4290 or write to:

> ArcVentures Medical Education Services
> 820 West Jackson Boulevard, Suite 750
> Chicago, IL 60607

National Medical School Review

National Medical School Review offers live-lecture review programs in preparation for any of the three USMLE examinations. Lecturers are faculty at US medical schools, and some instructors are also authors of Step 1 and Step 2 review books. Additionally, the courses offer testing workshops covering such topics as test-taking skills, cognitive skills, stress-reduction techniques, and faculty-led subject testing. Extensive written notes and several published review books are also provided.

National Medical School Review offers a variety of programs 3 to 13 weeks in length, depending upon the student's needs. The three-week course is designed for US medical students taking USMLE Step 1 for the first time. The seven-week Basic Science course offers a comprehensive review of material in

REVIEW RESOURCES

Commercial Courses

the basic sciences with particular attention to those areas highly represented on the exam. The six-week Clinical Science course provides instruction in clinical areas required to pass the USMLE Step 2 exam. The 13-week course in Basic Science is intended for students who require a more intensive comprehensive review. Diagnostic testing is featured at the start of each course, and results are interpreted under guidance of testing specialists.

Costs range from $1000 for the three-week program to $5000 for the 13-week program. The program sites include Atlanta, Illinois, New Jersey, and Southern California. Courses are scheduled throughout the year. To receive an application and more information, call (800) 533-8850 or (714) 476-6282 or write to:

National Medical School Review
4500 Campus Drive, Suite 201
Newport Beach, CA 92660

Northwestern Learning Center

Northwestern Learning Center offers live-lecture review camps in preparation for both the USMLE Steps 1 and 2, and the NBOME Parts 1 and 2 examinations. The programs utilize the TALLP methodology (*Test-Taking Application of Logic, Language, and Psychology*), which focuses on medical test-taking techniques and provides a system of choosing answers based on the logical structure and holistic patterns of board questions. Two programs are available: NBI 300 (*Intensive Care for the Boards*) and NBI 100 (*Primary Care for the Boards*). NBI 300 is offered in 15-day, 21-day, and 28-day review camp formats immediately prior to each scheduled National Board examination. NBI 300 courses include live lectures taught by faculty from various universities and/or authors of review board manuals, simulated exams, group study, and printed lecture notes. Review camps are held at resorts, convention centers, and universities throughout the country. Course costs range from $880 to $1750. NBI 100 is an on-site, one day workshop focusing on medical test-taking and TALLP techniques. It also assists students in organizing a self-study plan, applying memorization techniques, identifying high-impact subject areas, and learning about various board preparation resources. NBI 100 is available only to groups of students or contracting medical schools. The cost of NBI 100 ranges from $85 to $120 per student. For more information, call (800) 837-7737 or (517) 332-0777 or write to:

Northwestern Learning Center
4700 S. Hagadorn
East Lansing, MI 48823

Postgraduate Medical Review Education (PMRE)

PMRE offers a videotaped lecture series covering the basic sciences on a year-round basis in Miami Beach, Florida. Other course sites may be announced for 1996. Tuition ranges from $1000 for the "crash" course to $3500 for the full course. Books and audiotapes covering the basic sciences are also available. For more information call (800) 433-3539 or write to:

PMRE
407 Lincoln Rd., #12I
Miami Beach, FL 33139

The Princeton Review

The Princeton Review offers personalized workshops in the basic sciences for the USMLE Step 1 exam. In 1996, USMLE Step 1 courses will be offered in Boston, Chicago, Detroit, Dallas, Houston, Long Island, Los Angeles, Miami, New York, Philadelphia, San Francisco, and Washington DC. The Princeton Review is also offering programs on site at selected medical schools across the country in May. Courses for the Step 2 and 3 will also be offered in 1996. Course schedules and prices vary.

Students take a placement diagnostic exam and receive detailed feedback, recommendations for study, and tips for test taking in general. Based on the placement exam, students are then assigned to classes limited to 12 to 15 students per instructor. The course follows a traditional subject-based progression but employs small-group learning precepts instead of large-lecture formats. Each instructor scored in the top 20th percentile of the USMLE Step 1 exam. The small-group format and materials allow flexibility in meeting individual needs.

The Princeton Review provides extensive student workshop manuals and subject-specific content reference, all written by content experts and approved or revised by instructors who passed the exam. Extra tutoring is available. Lessons in each subject are reinforced with exams to assess strengths and weaknesses. A final review led by medical school faculty addresses any remaining knowledge gaps.

For more information, send e-mail to info.tpr@review.com, call 1-800-USMLE84 or write to:

The Princeton Review
2315 Broadway, Third Floor
New York, NY 10024

Kaplan Educational Center

Kaplan's comprehensive USMLE Step 1 course is a multi-modal, self-study program that is available throughout the year. With the help of diagnostic exams and computerized feedback, students are guided through the material and study at their own pace. Some students enroll in their first year of medical school so that they can use the program to supplement their regular coursework.

The Kaplan course includes a set of newly revised review books that focuses on the core basic science material tested, thousands of USMLE-style review questions grouped by subject area and organ system, subject area final exams, three-hour simulated exams with computerized feedback, and a complete set of lecture videos, taught by US medical school faculty, with accompanying handouts. A full course syllabus integrates all of the materials and provides study suggestions and test-taking strategies.

For 1996, Kaplan is introducing an intensive eight-week live-lecture program taught by US medical school faculty, in select locations. A bonus of four weeks of center access is included. Also available is Boards Express, a program exclusively for second-year medical students, which provides access to all of their library material in the last month before the exam.

There are over 100 Kaplan Medical centers nationwide and around the world. The price of the course varies with the length of study time. Discounts are available for Kaplan MCAT alumni. For more information call 1-800-KAP-TEST, or write to

Kaplan Medical
810 Seventh Avenue, 22nd Floor
New York, NY 10019

Youel's Prep, Inc.

Youel's Prep offers a live lecture-and-discussion test preparation program for the USMLE Steps 1, 2, and 3. The lectures are given by Dr. Youel at various sites and dates throughout the United States. The Step 1 course format is a one-week, eight-hour-per-day program with over 1,000 pages of Prep Notes and three test booklets. Tuition is $750; a group discount is available. An 18-day, $1500 program is also available. Students can repeat the course at no charge. In addition, the written notes can be purchased separately at $400 per set. New for 1996 is the $600 Youel's Study Program, which includes a comprehensive organ-system-based review, 3000 practice questions with explanations, and detailed reviews of study and testing strategies. For more information, call (800) 645-3985 or call collect (616) 795-9273 (if outside the US) or write to:

Youel's Prep, Inc.
P.O. Box 888-453
Grand Rapids, MI 49588-8453

Publisher Contacts

If you do not have convenient access to a medical bookstore, consider ordering directly from the publisher.

Appleton & Lange
P.O. Box 120041
Stamford, CT 06912
(800) 423-1359
Fax: (203) 406-4600/4602

Blackwell Scientific
238 Main Street
Cambridge, MA 02142
(800) 759-6102
Fax: (617) 876-7022

Churchill Livingstone
5 South 250 Frontenac Road
Naperville, IL 60563-1711
(800) 553-5426
Fax: (708) 983-5576

FMSG Inc.
P.O. Box 7471
Freeport, NY 11520
(800) 662-3244
Fax: (516) 826-8099

ILOC Inc.
P.O. Box 232
Granville, OH 43203
(800) 495-4562
(614) 587-2658
Fax: (614) 587-2679

J&S Publishing
1300 Bishop Lane
Alexandria, VA 22302
(703) 823-9833
Fax: (703) 823-9834
Jandspub@ix.netcom.com

Lippincott-Raven Publishers
P.O. Box 1580
Hagerstown, MD 21741
(800) 777-2295
Fax: (301) 824-7390

Little, Brown and Company
200 West Street
Waltham, MA 02154
(800) 343-9204
Fax: (617) 890-0875

McGraw-Hill Customer Service
860 Taylor Station Road
Blacklick, OH 43004
(800) 262-4729
Fax: (614) 759-3644

MedMaster, Inc.
P.O. Box 640028
Miami, FL 33164
(800) 335-3480
(305) 653-3480
Fax: (305) 653-9678
stgoldberg@aol.com

Michaelis Medical Publishing
2274 South 1300 East
Suite G8-288
Salt Lake City, UT 84106
(800) 557-6672
Fax: (801) 273-7707

Mosby-Year Book
11830 Westline Industrial Drive
St. Louis, MO 63146
(800) 325-4177 ext. 5017
Fax: (800) 535-9935
www.mosby.com

National Learning Corporation
212 Michael Drive
Syosset, NY 11791
(800) 645-6337
Fax: (516) 921-8743

Springer-Verlag, NY Inc.
Attention: Service Center
333 Meadowlands Parkway
Secaucus, NJ 07094
(800) 777-4643
Fax: (201) 348-5405
www.Springer-NY.com
orders@Springer-NY.com

W.B. Saunders
6277 Sea Harbor Drive
Orlando, FL 32887
(800) 545-2522

Williams & Wilkins
P.O. Box 1496
Baltimore, MD 21298-9724
(800) 638-0672
Fax: (800) 477-8438
www.wwilkins.com

Data in Section III were verified by Discount Medical Books & Supplies and Reiter's Professional Books—independent bookstores that are able to ship books from multiple publishers at list price both domestically and internationally.

Discount Medical Books & Supplies
345 Judah Street
San Francisco, CA 94122
(415) 664-5555
Fax: (415) 664-7810
Medicalme@aimnet.com

Reiter's Scientific & Professional Books
2021 K Street, N.W.
Washington, DC 20006-1003
(800) 537-4314
(202) 223-3327
Fax: (202) 296-9103
books@reiters.com

Abbreviations and Symbols

Abbreviation	Meaning	Abbreviation	Meaning
Ab	antibody	DPPC	dipalmitoylphosphatidylcholine
ACE	angiotensin-converting enzyme	ds	double stranded
ACh	acetylcholine	dTMP	deoxythymidine monophosphate
AD	autosomal dominant	DTR	deep tendon reflex
ADA	adenosine deaminase	DTs	delirium tremens
ADH	antidiuretic hormone	EBV	Epstein-Barr virus
Ag	antigen	ECF	extracellular fluid
AIDS	acquired immune deficiency syndrome	ECT	electroconvulsive therapy
ALA	aminolevulinate synthase	EDRF	endothelium-derived relaxing factor
ALL	acute lymphocytic leukemia	EDTA	ethylenediamine tetraacetic acid
AML	acute myelogenous leukemia	EDV	end-diastolic volume
ALS	amyotrophic lateral sclerosis	EEG	electroencephalogram
ALT	alanine transaminase	EF-2	elongation factor 2
ANA	antinuclear antibody	EGF	epidermal growth factor
ANP	atrial natriuretic peptide	EM	electron microscopy
ANS	autonomic nervous system	EMB	eosin-methylene blue
ARDS	acute respiratory distress syndrome	EPS	extrapyramidal symptoms
ASD	atrial septal defect	ER	endoplasmic reticulum; emergency room
ASO	antistreptolysin O	ERP	effective refractory period
AST	aspartate transaminase	ESR	erythrocyte sedimentation rate
AV	atrioventricular	ESV	end-systolic volume
AVM	arteriovenous malformation	EtOH	ethyl alcohol
AZT	azidothymidine	FAD	oxidized flavin adenine dinucleotide
BAL	British anti-Lewisite (dimercaprol)	$FADH_2$	reduced flavin adenine dinucleotide
BP	blood pressure	FEV	forced expiratory volume
BPG	bis phosphoglycerate	FF	filtration fraction
CAD	coronary artery disease	FFP	fresh frozen plasma
cAMP	cyclic adenosine monophosphate	FMN	flavin mononucleotide
CCK	cholecystokinin	FSH	follicle-stimulating hormone
CD	cluster of differentiation	FTA-ABS	fluorescent treponemal antibody—absorbed
CDC	Centers for Disease Control		
CDP	cytidine diphosphate	FVC	forced vital capacity
cGMP	cyclic guanosine monophosphate	G3P	glucose-3-phosphate
ChAT	choline acetyltransferase	G6PD	glucose-6-phosphate dehydrogenase
CHF	congestive heart failure	GABA	γ-aminobutyric acid
CJD	Creutzfeldt-Jakob disease	GFAP	glial fibrillary acidic protein
CML	chronic myelogenous leukemia	GFR	glomerular filtration rate
CMV	cytomegalovirus	G_i	G protein, inhibitory
CN	cranial nerve	GM-CSF	granulocyte-macrophage colony-stimulating factor
CO	cardiac output		
CoA	coenzyme A	GMP	guanosine monophosphate
COMT	catechol-O-methyltransferase	GN	glomerulonephritis
COPD	chronic obstructive pulmonary disease	GnRH	gonadotropin-releasing hormone
CPK-MB	creatine phosphokinase, MB fraction	G_s	G protein, stimulatory
CSF	cerebrospinal fluid	GTP	guanosine triphosphate
CT	computed tomography	Hb	hemoglobin
DAG	diacylglycerol	HAV	hepatitis A virus
DES	diethylstilbestrol	HBV	hepatitis B virus
DIC	disseminated intravascular coagulation	HCV	hepatitis C virus
DIMS	disorder in initiating and maintaining sleep	hCG	human chorionic gonadotropin
DMD	Duchenne muscular dystrophy	HDL	high-density lipoprotein
DMN	dorsal motor nucleus	HDV	hepatitis D virus
2,4-DNP	2,4-dinitrophenol	HEV	hepatitis E virus
DOES	disorder of excessive somnolence	HGPRT	hypoxanthine guanine-phosphoribosyltransferase
DPG	diffuse proliferative glomerulonephritis		
DPG	diphosphoglycerate	HLA	human leukocyte antigen

Abbreviation	Meaning
HMG	human menopausal gonadotropin
HMG-CoA	hydroxy-methyl-glutaryl CoA
HMP	hexose monophosphate
HPV	human papillomavirus
HSV	herpes simplex virus
HTLV	human T-cell lymphotropic virus
HTN	hypertension
ICF	intracellular fluid
IDL	intermediate-density lipoprotein
IFN	interferon
Ig	immunoglobulin
IHSS	idiopathic hypertrophic subaortic stenosis
IL-1	interleukin-1
IM	intramuscular
IMP	inosine monophosphate
IND	investigational new drug
INH	isonicotine hydrazine (isoniazid)
IP$_3$	inositol triphosphate
IVC	inferior vena cava
JGA	juxtaglomerular apparatus
LA	left atrium
LCAT	lecithin-cholesterol acyltransferase
LDH	lactate dehydrogenase
LDL	low-density lipoprotein
LFT	liver function test
LH	luteinizing hormone
LMN	lower motor neuron (signs)
LT	leukotriene
M-CSF	macrophage colony-stimulating factor
MAC	*Mycobacterium avium-intracellulare* complex
MAO	monoamine oxidase
MEN	multiple endocrine neoplasia
MHC	major histocompatibility complex
MPTP	1-methyl-4-phenyl-1, 2, 3, 6-tetrahydro-pyridine
MTP	metatarsal-phalangeal
NAD	oxidized nicotinamide adenine dinucleotide
NADH	reduced nicotinamide adenine dinucleotide
NADP	oxidized nicotinamide adenine dinucleotide phosphate
NADPH	reduced nicotinamide adenine dinucleotide phosphate
NE	norepinephrine
NREM	non–rapid eye movement
NSAID	nonsteroidal anti-inflammatory drug
OAA	oxaloacetic acid
OBS	organic brain syndrome
PABA	para-aminobenzoic acid
PAH	para-aminohippuric acid
PALS	periarterial lymphoid sheath
PAN	polyarteritis nodosa
PAS	periodic acid–Schiff (stain)
PCI$_2$	prostacyclin I$_2$
PCAT	phosphatidylcholine-cholesterol acyltransferase
PCP	Pneumocystis carinii pneumonia
PCR	polymerase chain reaction
PDA	patent ducus arteriosus
PDE	phosphodiesterase
PDGF	platelet-derived growth factor
PEP	phosphoenolpyruvate
PFK	phosphofructokinase
PGE	prostaglandin E
PID	pelvic inflammatory disease
PIP$_2$	phosphatidylinositol 4,5-biphosphate
PKU	phenylketonuria

Abbreviation	Meaning
PML	progressive multifocal leukoencephalopathy
PMN	polymorphonuclear
PNH	paroxysmal nocturnal hemoglobinuria
PNS	peripheral nervous system
POMC	pro-opiomelanocortin
PP	pyrophosphate
PPRF	parapontine reticular formation
PRPP	phosphoribosylpyrophosphate
PSA	prostate-specific antigen
PT	prothrombin time
PTT	partial thromboplastin time
PTH	parathyroid hormone
RA	right atrium
REM	rapid eye movement
RES	reticuloendothelial system
RPF	renal plasma flow
RSV	respiratory syncytial virus
RVH	right ventricular hypertrophy
SA	sino-atrial
SAM	*S*-adenosylmethionine
SC	sickle cell, subcutaneous
SCID	severe combined immunodeficiency disease
SEM	standard error of the mean
SES	socioeconomic status
SGOT	serum glutamic oxaloacetic transaminase
SGPT	serum glutamic pyruvic transaminase
SLE	systemic lupus erythematosus
SRS-A	slow-reacting substance of anaphylaxis
ss	single stranded
SSPE	subacute sclerosing panencephalitis
SV	stroke volume
TAT	thematic apperception test
TB	tuberculosis
TCA	tricarboxylic acid
TGV	transposition of great vessels
TLC	total lung capacity
TNF	tissue necrosis factor
TPP	thiamine pyrophosphate
TSH	thyroid-stimulating hormone
TxA$_2$	thromboxane A$_2$
UDP	uridine diphosphate
UMN	upper motor neuron (signs)
URI	upper respiratory infection
UTI	urinary tract infection
VDRL	Venereal Disease Research Laboratory
VF	ventricular fibrillation
V/Q	ratio of ventilation to perfusion
VLDL	very low-density lipoprotein
VMA	vanillylmandelic acid
VSD	ventricular septal defect
VZV	varicella zoster virus

Symbol	Meaning
↑	increase(s)
↓	decrease(s)
→	leads to
1°	primary
2°	secondary
3°	tertiary
≈	approximately; homologous
≡	defined as

Index

PAS stain, 51
Patau's syndrome, 135
Patent ductus arteriosus, 135
Pathology
    high-yield facts, 133–160
    review resources for, 247–250
Pectinate line, 51
Pelvic inflammatory disease, 119
Penicillin, 162
    and gram-negative bugs, 111
Penile abnormalities, congenital, 46
Pentamidine, 166
Pentavalent antimony, 166
Pentose phosphate pathway, 91
PEP carboxylase, 91
Pepsin, secretion of, 207
Pericarditis, 152
Perilymph, 52
Peripheral nerve layers, 52
Peripheral nervous system, supportive cells, 56
Periplasmic space, 111
Personality disorders, 76
    cluster A, 76
    cluster B, 76
    cluster C, 76
Pertussis toxins, 113
Peyer's patch, 55
Pharmacokinetics, 192
Pharmacology
    high-yield facts, 161–194
    high-yield topics, 193
    review resources for, 251–253
Pharyngeal pouch, derivatives of, 45
Phase II metabolism, 192
Phase I metabolism, 192
Phenotypic mixing, 121
Phenoxybenzamine, 169
Phentolamine, 169
Phenylephrine, 168
Phenylketonuria, 88
Phenytoin, 171
Pheochromocytoma, 142
Phobia(s), 75, 77
    social, 75
Phosphatidylcholine, function of, 98
Physiology
    high-yield facts, 71–72, 195–216
    review resources for, 255–257
Physostigmine, 167
Piaget, Jean, stages of development, 70
Pick's disease, 146
Picornavirus, 124
Pilocarpine, 167
PIP₂ second messenger system, 99
Pituitary glycoprotein hormones, 212
Plasia definitions, 138
Plasma membrane, composition of, 98
Pneumocystis carinii, 117
Polio, 146
Polyadenylation, 86
Polycystic kidney disease
    in adults, 137
    in childhood, 136
Polymerase chain reaction, 85
Polymerases
    DNA, 85
    RNA, 85
Polymyxins, 165
Pompe's disease, 88
Portal-systemic anastomoses, 50
Posterior pituitary, 55
Postgraduate Medical Review Education, 261
Posttraumatic stress disorder, 76
Potassium channel blockers, 178
Potter's syndrome, 47
Power, 66
Praziquantel, 166
Prazosin, 169, 173
Precancerous conditions, 139
Precipitin curve, 127
Precision, versus accuracy, 65
Predictive value, 64
Prednisone, 181
Preload, 197
Premature infants, 67

Pressure, 198
Prevalence, versus incidence, 64
Princeton Review, 262
Prions, 121
Progesterone, 214
Progressive systemic sclerosis, 148
Projection, 78
Projective tests, 77
Propylthiouracil, 190
Protein, 103
    high-yield facts, 97–99
Protein synthesis
    ATP versus GTP, 95
    direction of, 95
Protein synthesis inhibitors, 163
Prussian blue stain, 51
Psammoma bodies, 156
Pseudocyst, 46
Pseudohermaphrodite
    female, 135
    male, 135
Pseudomonas aeruginosa, 112
Psychiatry, 81
    cultural/ethnic, 73
    forensic, 73
    high-yield facts, 73–78
Psychoanalysis, 79
    existential, 79
    topography in, 79
Psychology, 81
    high-yield facts, 78–80
Psychosis, Schneiderian signs of, 77
Pudendal nerve block, landmarks for, 51
Pulmonary circulation, 204
Pulmonary physiology, 215
Pyridostigmine, 167
Pyridoxine, 100
Pyruvate carboxylase, 91
Pyruvate dehydrogenase complex, 92
Pyruvate dehydrogenase deficiency, 87

Q
Quinine, 166

R
Rabies virus, 125
Radial nerve, 47
    injury to, 48
Rationalization, 78
Reaction formation, 78
Reassortment, 121
Recombination, 121
Recurrent laryngeal nerve, 48
Red blood cell(s). *See also* Erythrocyte(s)
    energetics, 93
    forms, 156
Reflex arc, 59
Regression, 78
    in children, 70
Reinforcement schedules, 79
Reiter's syndrome, 148
Relative risk, 64
Reliability, 65
REM rebound, 72
REM sleep, 72
Renal clearance, 208
Renal failure, 209
Renal physiology, 215
    high-yield facts, 208–211
Renal plasma flow, effective, 208
Renin-angiotensin system, 210
Reportable diseases, 67
Repression, 78
Reproductive physiology, 215
Reserpine, 173
Resistance, 198
Respiratory physiology, high-yield facts, 203–205
Restrictive lung disease, 205
Reticular activating system, lesions of, 57
Retinol, 99
Retired NBME Basic Medical Sciences (Part I) Test Items, 8–10
Review resources, 217–258
    for anatomy, 227–233
    for behavioral science, 235–236

for biochemistry, 237–240
for microbiology, 241–245
for pathology, 247–250
for pharmacology, 251–253
for physiology, 255–257
Reye's syndrome, 149
Rheumatic fever, 152
Rheumatic heart disease, 152
Rheumatic pathology, 158
    high-yield facts, 147–149
Rheumatoid arthritis, 147
Rhizopus species, 117
Riboflavin, 100
Rickettsiae, 114
Rickettsial diseases, 114
    vectors of, 114
Rifampin, 165
Right parietal lobe, lesions of, 57
Ritodrine, 186
RNA, 103
    high-yield facts, 84–86
    processing of, 86
    synthesis direction, 85
    types of, 86
RNA polymerases, 85
RNA viral strands, 120
RNA viruses
    enveloped, 124
    nonenveloped, 124
Rocky Mountain spotted fever, 114
Rods, 42
Rotator cuff muscles, 50
Rotavirus, 124
Roth's spots, 156
Rough endoplasmic reticulum, 53
Rule of 2's for 2nd week of development, 43

S
S-adenosyl-methionine, 90
Salivary secretion, 206
Salmonella, versus *Shigella*, 113
Sarcoidosis, 148
Scalp, layers of, 48
Schizophrenia, 77
    neurotransmitter changes in, 71
Schneiderian signs of psychosis, 77
Schwann cells, 42, 56
Scleroderma, 148
Scopolamine, 167
Secretin, secretion of, 207
Secretion, types of, 54
Segmented viruses, 124
Selective immunoglobulin deficiency, 130
Selegiline, 170
Self-Test in the Part I Basic Medical Sciences, 8–10
Sensitivity, 64
Sensory deprivation effects, 72
Sentinel loop, 157
Sentinel node, 157
Serotonin reuptake inhibitors, 170
Severe combined immunodeficiency, 89, 130
Sexual dysfunction, 80
Sexual response, male, autonomic innervation of, 51
Shigella, versus *Salmonella*, 113
Sickle cell anemia, 138
Sick role, 78
Signal molecule precursors, 97
Silver stain, 51
Sinus, 46
Sinusoids
    of liver, 54
    of spleen, 54
Sjögren's syndrome, 149
Skeletal muscle, versus cardiac, electrophysiological differences, 200
Skew distribution, 65
Sleep patterns, in depressed patients, 72
Sleep stages, 72
Slow viruses, 121
Smooth endoplasmic reticulum, 54
Social phobia, 75
Socioeconomic status, Hollingshead determinants of, 66